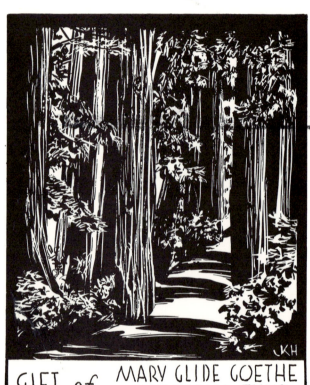

GIFT of MARY GLIDE GOETHE
MEMORIAL FUND

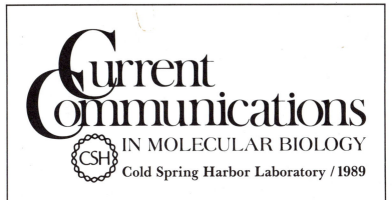

Cytoskeletal
Proteins in
Tumor Diagnosis

Edited by

Mary Osborn
Max-Planck Institute for Biophysical Chemistry

Klaus Weber
Max-Planck Institute for Biophysical Chemistry

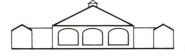

A Banbury Center Meeting

CYTOSKELETAL PROTEINS IN TUMOR DIAGNOSIS
Copyright 1989 by Cold Spring Harbor Laboratory
All rights reserved
International Standard Book Number 0-87969-325-8
Book design by Emily Harste
Printed in the United States of America

Cover: (*Left*) Human breast carcinoma cell line MCF7, x250; (*middle*) histological section of human mammary carcinoma, x160; (*right*) aspiration cytology of human primary mammary carcinoma, x250. All stained with antibodies to keratin in indirect immunofluorescence microscopy. All tumor cells are keratin-positive. (Courtesy Drs. M. Osborn, M. Altmannsberger, and W. Domagala.)

The individual summaries contained herein should not be treated as publications or listed in bibliographies. Information contained herein can be cited as personal communication contingent upon obtaining the consent of the author. The collected work may, however, be cited as a general source of information on this topic.

All Cold Spring Harbor Laboratory publications may be ordered directly from Cold Spring Harbor Laboratory, Box 100, Cold Spring Harbor, New York 11724. (Phone: Continental U.S. except New York State 1-800-843-4388. All other locations [516] 367-8325.)

Conference Participants

Michael Altmannsberger, Dept. of Pathology, University of Giessen, Federal Republic of Germany

Susan P. Banks-Schlegel, Division of Lung Diseases, NHLB Institute, National Institutes of Health, Bethesda, Maryland

Hector Battifora, Division of Pathology, City of Hope National Medical Center, Duarte, California

Nicholas J. Cowan, Dept. of Biochemistry, New York University Medical Center, New York

Pamela Cowin, Dept. of Cell Biology and Dermatology, New York University School of Medicine, New York

Bruce A. Cunningham, Dept. of Developmental and Molecular Biology, Rockefeller University, New York, New York

Ivan Damjanov, Dept. of Pathology and Cell Biology, Jefferson Medical College of Thomas Jefferson University, Philadelphia, Pennsylvania

Werner W. Franke, Institute of Cell and Tumor Biology, German Cancer Research Center, Heidelberg, Federal Republic of Germany

Giulio Gabbiani, Dept. of Pathology, CMU, University of Geneva, Switzerland

Kevin C. Gatter, Nuffield Dept. of Pathology, John Radcliffe Hospital, Oxford, England

Adi F. Gazdar, NCI-Navy Medical Oncology Branch, National Cancer Institute and Naval Hospital, Bethesda, Maryland

Victor E. Gould, Dept of Pathology, Rush-Presbyterian-St. Luke's Medical Center, Chicago, Illinois

Allen M. Gown, Dept. of Pathology, University of Washington, Seattle

David Helfman, Cold Spring Harbor Laboratory, Cold Spring Harbor, New York

Harriette Kahn, Dept. of Pathology, Women's College Hospital, Toronto, Canada

Leopold G. Koss, Dept. of Pathology, Montefiore Medical Center and Albert Einstein College of Medicine, Bronx, New York

C. Chandra Kumar, Dept. of Tumor Biology, Schering Research Corporation, Bloomfield, New Jersey

Birgitte Lane, Imperial Cancer Research Fund, Clare Hall Laboratories, Hertfordshire, England

Daniel Louvard, Dept. of Molecular Biology, Institut Pasteur, Paris, France

Markku Miettinen, Dept. of Pathology, University of Helsinki, Finland

Roland Moll, Institute of Pathology, University of Mainz, Federal Republic of Germany

Jon S. Morrow, Dept. of Pathology, Yale University School of Medicine, New Haven, Connecticut

Ray B. Nagle, Dept. of Pathology, University of Arizona, Tucson

Mary Osborn, Max-Planck-Institute for Biophysical Chemistry, Goettingen, Federal Republic of Germany

Frans Ramaekers, Dept. of Pathology, University Hospital, Nijmegen, The Netherlands

James G. Rheinwald, Division of Cell Growth and Regulation, Dana-Farber Cancer Institute, Boston, Massachusetts

Gert Riethmüller, Institute of Immunology, University of Munich, Federal Republic of Germany

Dennis R. Roop, Dept. of Health and Human Services, National Institutes of Health, Bethesda, Maryland

Michael L. Shelanski, Dept. of Pathology and Center for Neurobiology and Behavior, Columbia University College of Physicians & Surgeons, New York, New York

Ludwig A. Sternberger, Dept. of Neurology, Anatomy, and Pathology, University of Maryland School of Medicine, Baltimore, Maryland

Tung-Tien Sun, Dept. of Dermatology and Pharmacology, New York University Medical Center, New York

John Q. Trojanowski, Dept. of Pathology and Laboratory Medicine, University of Pennsylvania School of Medicine, Philadelphia

Ismo Virtanen, Dept. of Anatomy, University of Helsinki, Finland

Arthur M. Vogel, Dept. of Pathology, St. Louis University Medical Center, Missouri

Preface

Most cytoskeletal proteins belong to multigene families, which show distinct cell- and tissue-specific expression patterns. This situation for the six different actins was first seen by protein sequencing, whereas for tubulins, cDNA sequencing and use of peptide antibodies were necessary to establish the different distributions of the tubulin isoforms. The knowledge accumulated about the expression of intermediate filament proteins has shown that they are particularly valuable markers of cell lineage. Other cytoskeletal proteins of potential use in cell typing discussed in this volume include chain-specific keratin antibodies, desmoplakins, spectrins, tropomyosins, synaptophysin, and villin. None of these proteins are tumor antigens, but as markers of cell type and of differentiated state, they all deserve attention.

We welcomed the chance to bring together cell and molecular biologists and practicing pathologists under the auspices of the Banbury Center of Cold Spring Harbor Laboratory. These abstracts summarize the state of the art in October 1988. They emphasize both the expression rules followed by intermediate filament polypeptides and other cytoskeletal proteins in embryogenesis and in the adult mammal and the potential use and inherent limitations of antibodies to such proteins as markers of tumor type in human pathology.

We are grateful to those who made the meeting possible: Dr. Terri Grodzicker, who initiated the discussions, Dr. Jan Witkowski and Bea Toliver at the Banbury Center, who took over the organization of the meeting and were in large part responsible for its success, and Katya Davey, who as hostess of Robertson House made us all welcome. Thanks also to Nancy Ford (Managing Director of Publications), Dorothy Brown, Nadine Dumser, and Joan Ebert who produced and published this volume. We thank the James S. McDonnell Foundation for financial support of this meeting.

M.O.
K.W.

Contents

Regulation of Expression of the Gene Encoding Glial Filament Acidic Protein

S. Sarkar and N.J. Cowan

Department of Biochemistry, NYU Medical Center
New York, New York 10016

Available evidence indicates that differences in the expression of tissue-specific traits among various cells are largely a consequence of transcriptional regulation of corresponding gene sequences. In general, the regulation of gene expression is mediated by the interaction of adjacent DNA sequences and *trans*-acting factors (Dynan and Tijan 1985; Gluzman 1985). Studies of viral (Hen et al. 1982; Miyamoto et al. 1984) and eukaryotic (Banerjee et al. 1983; Gillies et al. 1983) genes have revealed the presence of a number of distinct transcriptional control elements, including the TATA box, upstream promoter elements, enhancers, and silencers, located upstream or downstream from the transcription initiation site. These sequences act in *cis* to regulate transcriptional initiation by RNA polymerase II. More recently, proteins that specifically bind to these *cis*-acting DNA elements have been identified by in vitro DNA-binding assays (Carthew et al. 1985).

We have focused our attention on the expression and regulation of genes that are selectively expressed in the mammalian central nervous system (CNS). The mammalian CNS is extremely complex in both cytoarchitecture and function. It has been estimated that about 30,000 mRNA species are expressed in brain, of which between 55% and 95% are brain-specific. This enormous complexity entails the transcriptional activity of 45% of the genome, and the great diversity of cell types and interconnections that are characteristic of the mammalian brain is, at least in part, a consequence of the complex spatial and temporal patterns of expression of these genes.

Glial fibrillary acidic protein (GFAP), the principal component of glial filaments, is notable in that it represents a specific marker for the astroglial cells in the mammalian CNS (Bignami et al. 1972). A cloned cDNA probe encoding mouse GFAP has been isolated (Lewis et al. 1984). This probe has been used for the isolation and structural characterization of

1

the corresponding single-copy gene (Balcarek and Cowan 1985). The entire sequence of the mouse GFAP gene totaling 9.8 kb has been determined. However, the molecular basis for the tissue-restricted expression of GFAP is completely unknown.

We report here the detection of a *cis*-acting sequence of approximately 40 nucleotides, which regulates the expression of the GFAP gene. The approach was to generate progressive deletions of GFAP promoter upstream sequences, followed by transfection into GFAP-expressing and nonexpressing cells. We also report the use of an electrophoretic mobility-shift assay (Carthew et al. 1985) to define the interaction of a factor or factors with sequences in this region.

RESULTS
Localization of a *cis*-Acting Element by Upstream Deletion Analysis of the Mouse GFAP Gene
To delimit sequences essential for the expression of the mouse GFAP gene, we constructed a series of deletion mutants in the 5' -flanking region. The transcriptional capacity of these deletion mutants was assayed by RNase protection (Melton et al. 1984), following transfection into the GFAP-producing cell line U251 or into a nonexpressing human epithelial cell line (HeLa). A protected band of about 230 nucleotides resulting from correctly initiated transcripts was found only in GFAP-producing U251 cells. Deletion of sequences upstream of –107 does not affect the level of expression, whereas deletion of sequence between –107 and –94 causes a slight reduction in the level of transcription. Further deletion to –78 results in a drastic reduction in transcription of the mouse GFAP gene in U251 cells.

Similar results were obtained with a rat glioma cell line (C6), which expresses GFAP at a very low, but nevertheless detectable, level. We conclude that U251 and C6 glioma cells both contain protein factors that interact with *cis*-acting DNA sequences in the –107 to –78 region to switch on the GFAP gene in these cell lines, whereas nonexpressing HeLa cells either lack the positive *trans*-acting factor or contain repressors that inhibit the expression of GFAP.

Identification of a Protein Factor That Binds to the *cis*-Acting Regulatory Element
We have used an electrophoretic mobility-shift assay to identify protein factor(s) binding to the DNA sequence shown to be es-

2

sential for the expression of the GFAP gene. When a 40-bp fragment extending from −107 to −67 was labeled at the 5′ end and incubated with a crude nuclear extract prepared from either U251, C6, or HeLa cells, a band with reduced mobility was detected on a nondenaturing polyacrylamide gel. This band was readily competed out by unlabeled fragment but not by nonspecific DNA, e.g., pUC or increasing amounts of poly(dI-dC).

Precise Localization by DNase I Protection of the Binding Site Recognized by a Protein Factor

To achieve a precise localization of this transcription factor on upstream GFAP DNA, we have used DNase I footprinting analysis (Galas and Schmitz 1978; Landolfi et al. 1987). The regions between nucleotide −97 and −80 on the noncoding strand and between −100 and −81 on the coding strand were protected from DNase I digestion. However, the protection on the coding strand seems to be somewhat weaker than that on the noncoding strand.

DISCUSSION

Transfection experiments showed that introduced DNA sequences encoding mouse GFAP can be expressed in cells that are glial in origin (e.g., U251 and C6) but not in nonhomologous cells such as fibroblasts. This suggests either the presence of an activator or the absence of a repressor in homologous cells. The fact that identical band patterns were observed in all mobility-shift assays using both GFAP-expressing and non-expressing cell lines suggests the binding of some ubiquitous transcription factor. It seems possible that a second transcription factor specific to GFAP-expressing cells might bind to this ubiquitous factor, thereby activating the transcription of the gene. Further experiments are planned to test this hypothesis.

Our current efforts are directed toward a parallel analysis of the factors involved in the tissue-specific expression of the genes encoding the neurofilament proteins–intermediate filaments whose expression is restricted to neuronal cells.

REFERENCES

Balcarek, J.M. and N.J. Cowan. 1985. Structure of the mouse glial fibrillary acidic protein gene: Implications for the evolution of the intermediate filament multigene family. *Nucleic Acids Res.* **13:** 5527.
Banerjee, J., L. Olson, and W. Shaffner. 1983. Lymphocyte specific cel-

lular enhancer is located downstream of the joining region in the immunoglobulin heavy chain gene. *Cell* **33:** 729.

Bignami, A., L.F. Eng, D. Dahl, and C.T. Dyeda. 1972. Localization of the glial fibrillary acidic protein in astrocytes by immunofluorescence. *Brain Res.* **43:** 429.

Carthew, R.W., L.A. Chodosh, and P.A. Sharp. 1985. An RNA polymerase II transcription factor binds to an upstream domain in the adenovirus major late promoter. *Cell* **43:** 439.

Dynan, W.S. and R. Tjian. 1985. Control of eukaryotic messenger RNA synthesis by sequence specific DNA binding proteins. *Nature* **316:** 774.

Galas, D. and A. Schmitz. 1978. DNase footprinting — A simple method for the detection of protein DNA binding specificity. *Nucleic Acids Res.* **5:** 3157.

Gillies, S.D., S.L. Morrison, V.T. Oi, and S. Tonegawa. 1983. A tissue specific transcription enhancer element is located in the major intron of a rearranged immunoglobin heavy chain gene. *Cell* **33:** 717.

Gluzman, Y. 1985. *Current communications in molecular biology. Eukaryotic transcription: The role of cis and trans-acting elements in initiation.* Cold Spring Harbor Laboratory. Cold Spring Harbor, New York.

Hen, R., P. Sassone-Corsi, J. Corder, M.P. Gaub, and P. Chambon. 1982. Sequences upstream of TATA box are required in vivo and in vitro for efficient transcription from the adenovirus serotype II major late promoter. *Proc. Natl. Acad. Sci.* **79:** 7132.

Landolfi, N.F., J.D. Capra, and P.W. Tucker. 1987. Protein-nucleotide contacts in the immunoglobin heavy chain promoter regions. *Proc. Natl. Acad. Sci.* **84:** 3851.

Lewis, S.A., J.M. Balcarek, V. Krek, M.L. Shelanski, and N.J. Cowan. 1984. Sequence of a cDNA clone encoding glial fibrillary acidic protein: Structural conservation of intermediate filaments. *Proc. Natl. Acad. Sci.* **81:** 2743.

Melton, D.A., P.A. Kreig, M.R. Rebagliati, T. Maniatis, K. Zinn, and M.R. Green. 1984. Efficient in vitro synthesis of biologically active RNA and RNA hybridization probes from plasmids containing a bacteriophage SP6 promoter. *Nucleic Acids Res.* **12:** 7035.

Miyamoto, N., G. Moncollin, M. Wintzeritz, R. Hen, J.M. Egly, and P. Chambon. 1984. Stimulation of in vitro transcription by the upstream element of adenovirus II major later promoter involves a specific factor. *Nucleic Acids Res.* **12:** 8779.

Neurofilament Phosphorylation: Reactive and Degenerative

L.A. Sternberger,[1] H. Zhang,[1] L.J. Rubinstein,[2] M.M. Herman,[2] L.I. Binder,[3] and N.H. Sternberger[1]

[1]Departments of Neurology, Anatomy, and Pathology
University of Maryland School of Medicine
Baltimore, Maryland 21201

[2]Department of Pathology, University of Virginia
School of Medicine, Charlottesville, Virginia 22908

[3]Department of Anatomy, University of Alabama
School of Medicine, Birmingham, Alabama 35294

Neurofilaments consist of three proteins, NFL (light, 60 kD), NFM (medium, 160 kD), and NFH (heavy, 200 kD). NFL forms the core of the neurofilament structure, whereas segments of NFM and NFH are inserted into the core via a molecular region fairly close to their amino-terminal end. The relatively large carboxy-terminal ends of NFH and NFM protrude from the core in the form of whiskers. Julien and Mushinski (1983) have shown that NFH is generally phosphorylated heavily, whereas NFM is moderately phosphorylated and NFL is largely non-phosphorylated.

Our work on normal and pathologic neurofilaments has been the result of earlier investigations in the search for new proteins specific for individual neurons or individual groups of neurons. We produced a large number of monoclonal antibodies to whole brain homogenate and selected among the many antibody-producing hybridomas only those that stained, in formalin-fixed paraffin sections, given structures in brain without reacting even to minimal degrees with other structures in brain or any nonneuronal structures in peripheral tissues. Background-free immunocytochemistry, as provided by the unlabeled antibody ClonoPAP technique (Sternberger et al. 1970; Sternberger 1986), was essential for this purpose because background due to antibodies rather than the immunocytochemical method was a reason for rejection of hybridomas. Some of the more interesting monoclonal antibodies that came forth from this approach were specific for cilia (Sternberger et al. 1982), blood brain barrier (Sternberger and Sternberger 1987), and synaptic proteins (Sternberger et al. 1982), whereas a large group reacted with axons but not with neuronal cell bodies or dendrites. Antibodies of this group were found to react with NFH on immunoblots. Another group of monoclonal antibodies reacted with neuronal cell bodies and dendrites and only selected axons. To our surprise, these antibodies reacted with the NFH band on immunoblots as well. To solve this apparent paradox, we assumed that our monoclonal antibodies detected a posttranslational change in neurofilaments. During investigations on the nature of this change (Sternberger and Sternberger 1983), we found that axon-reactive antibodies bound to phosphorylated neurofilaments (PNfs), whereas cell body and dendrite-reactive antibodies bound to nonphosphorylated neurofilaments (nPNfs). Evidence for this conclusion was derived from haptane inhibition, two-dimensional electrophoresis of immunoreactive NFH, and effects of phosphatase on immunoreactivity. Each anti-PNf was apparently specific for a different conformation within or near the phosphorylation repeat segments of NFH. Anti-nPNf also exhibited heterogeneity of immunocytochemical distribution, and, indeed, some of them were found to be phosphorylation-dependent as they reacted only with nPNf and not with PNf. Other anti-nPNfs were phosphorylation-independent as they reacted with both nPNf and PNf. In tissue sections, immunostaining of anti-PNf was abolished by phosphatase pretreatment but not by trypsin pretreatment. Reaction of phosphorylation-dependent anti-PNf was unaffected by phosphatase but abolished by trypsin pretreatment. If trypsin treatment was followed by phosphatase, staining was restored, but the cell body-dendrite staining pattern had been converted to an axonal pattern, indicating unmasking of nonphosphorylated epitopes by dephosphorylation. Phosphorylation-independent anti-nPNfs were unaffected by treatment with phosphatase, only partially affected by treatment with trypsin, and unaffected by phosphatase after trypsin treatment.

Although perikaryonal neurofilaments were normally found free of phosphoepitopes in the central nervous system (Sternberger and Sternberger 1983), perikaryonal neurofilament phosphorylation was a common feature of a large variety of neurodegenerative disorders (Bizzi and Gambetti 1986; Forno et al. 1986; Howland and Alli 1986; Savita et al. 1986; Sima et al. 1986; Shiurba et al. 1987,1988). It also occurred after acute injury to the peripheral nerve (Rosenfeld et al. 1987) or spinal cord (Sternberger et al. 1989). In all of these cases, phosphorylation was detected by any of the available anti-PNfs and, therefore, might be considered a reactive process. An exception was found in Alzheimer's disease, where only one phosphoepitope has been regularly detected in perikaryonal tangles, leading to the concept that neurofilaments are abnormally processed in Alzheimer's disease (Sternberger et al. 1985; Cork et al. 1986). However, the very presence of neurofilaments in tangles has been questioned because of a reported cross-reaction of PNf with τ (Kiezak-Reding et al. 1987; Nukina et al. 1987). Because abnormal phosphorylation of τ is another feature of tangles, as reported by Grundke-Iqbal et al. (1986), the abnormal phosphorylation of neurofilaments could be questioned as well.

Even though Gambetti et al. (1987) and Cork et al. (1988) were unable to confirm the cross-reaction between τ and neurofilaments, we decided to reinvestigate it and found that four monoclonal anti-nPNfs and four monoclonal antibodies to PNf failed to react with τ. A fifth anti-PNf (07-5) cross-reacted with denatured τ at an affinity 1/1700 of that for denatured neurofilaments. Nondenatured τ in tissue sections did not cross-react. A fifth anti-nPNf (02-40) also cross-reacted weakly. All anti-PNfs, as well as anti-τ stained normal axons in Alzheimer's disease. Anti-nPNf failed to react with axons. Upon dephosphorylation, PNf staining disappeared, τ staining remained unchanged, and nPNf staining appeared in axons. Only one out of five anti-PNfs (07-5) stained nondephosphorylated tangles and only three stained plaques. These structures were not stained with anti-nPNf and only occasionally with anti-τ. Upon dephosphorylation, PNf staining disappeared and staining of tangles became prominent with anti-τ and generally with only one anti-nPNf (10-1); however, in plaques, staining with anti-τ and three anti-nPNfs became apparent. Quantitative data have shown that neurofilaments are indeed constituents of tangles, apparently exceeding the amount of τ 17-fold. Contribution of both conformation and primary structure to the specificity of IgG may be responsible for the absence of any cross-reaction of anti-neurofilaments with τ in intact tissue and its appearance in immunoblots in which contribution of con-

7

formation to specificity may be largely lost. The data extend earlier findings of abnormal processing of neurofilaments (Sternberger et al. 1985; Cork et al. 1986) and of τ (Grundke-Iqbal et al. 1986) in Alzheimer's disease and, taken together with reported abnormal processing of β-protein as well, as reported by Glenner (1988) and Allsop et al. (1988), may suggest that inhibition of processing of multiple proteins may be basic to the pathology of Alzheimer's disease; however, formation of plaques and tangles may merely be epiphenomena.

ACKNOWLEDGMENTS

This work was supported by U.S. Public Health Service grants (NS-24423, NS-26583, and NS-24185), a National Science Foundation grant (BNS-86-96080), and a grant from the State of Maryland.

REFERENCES

Allsop, D., C.W. Wong, S.-I. Ikeda, M.K. Landon, and C.G. Glenner. 1988. Immunohistochemical evidence for the derivation of a peptide ligand from the amyloid β-protein precursor of Alzheimer disease. *Proc. Natl. Acad. Sci.* **85**: 2790.

Bizzi, A. and P. Gambetti. 1986. Phosphorylation of neurofilaments is altered in aluminum intoxication. *Acta Neuropathol.* **71**: 154.

Cork, L.C., N.H. Sternberger, L.A. Sternberger, M.F. Casanova, R.G. Struble, and D.L. Price. 1986. Phosphorylated neurofilament antigens in neurofibrillary tangles in Alzheimer's disease. *J. Neuropathol. Exp. Neurol.* **45**: 56.

Cork., L.C., J.C. Troncoso, G.G. Klavano, E.S. Johnson, L.A. Sternberger, N.H. Sternberger, and D.L. Price. 1988. Neurofilament abnormalities in motor neurons in spontaneously occurring animal disorders. *J. Neuropathol. Exp. Neurol.* **47**: 420.

Forno, L.S., L.A. Sternberger, N.H. Sternberger, M.A. Strefling, K. Swanson, and L.F. Eng. 1986. Reaction of Lewy bodies with antibodies to phosphorylated and non-phosphorylated neurofilaments. *Neurosci. Lett.* **64**: 253.

Gambetti, P., L. Autilio-Gambetti, V. Manetto, and G. Perry. 1987. Composition of paired helical filaments of Alzheimer's disease as determined by specific probes. *Banbury Rep.* **27**: 309.

Glenner, G.G. 1988. Alzheimer's disease: Its proteins and genes. *Cell* **52**: 307.

Gold, B.G., J.W. Griffin, P.N. Hoffman, J. Rosenfeld, N.H. Sternberger, L.A. Sternberger, and D.L. Price. 1988. Neurofilament antigens in acrylamide neuropathy. *J. Neuropathol. Exp. Neurol.* **47**: 145.

Grundke-Iqbal, I., K. Iqbal, Y.-C. Tung, and N. Quinlin. 1986. Abnormal phosphorylation of the microtubule associated protein tau in Alzheimer cytoskeletal pathology. *Proc.Natl. Acad. Sci.* **83**: 4913.

Howland, R.D. and P. Alli. 1986. Altered phosphorylation of rat neuronal cytoskeletal proteins in acrylamide-induced neuropathy. *Brain Res.* 363: 333.

Julien, J.P. and W.E. Mushinski. 1983. The distribution of phosphorylation sites among identified proteolytic fragments of mammalian neurofilaments. *J. Biol. Chem.* 258: 4019.

Kiezak-Reding, H., D.W. Dickson, P. Davies, and S.-H. Yen. 1987. Recognition of tau epitopes by antineurofilament antibodies that bind to Alzheimer neurofibrillary tangles. *Proc. Natl. Acad. Sci.* 84: 3410.

Nukina, N., K. Kosik, and D. Selkoe. 1987. Recognition of Alzheimer paired helical filaments by monoclonal neurofilament antibodies is due to cross-reaction with tau protein. *Proc. Natl. Acad. Sci.* 84: 3415.

Rosenfeld, J., M.E. Dorman, J.W. Griffin, L.A. Sternberger, N.H. Sternberger, and D.L. Price. 1987. Distribution of neurofilament antigens after axonal injury. *J. Neuropathol. Exp. Neurol.* 46: 269.

Savita, E., D.M. Lapadula, and M.B. Abon-Donia. 1986. Calcium and calmodulin-enhanced in vitro phosphorylation of hen brain cold-stable microtubules and spinal cord neurofilament triplet proteins after a single oral dose of tri-o-cresyl phosphate. *Proc. Natl. Acad. Sci.* 83: 6174.

Shiurba, R.A., L.F. Eng, N.H. Sternberger, L.A. Sternberger, and H. Ulrich. 1987. The cytoskeleton of the human cerebellar cortex: An immunohistochemical study of normal and pathological material. *Brain Res.* 407: 208.

Shiurba, R.A., E.C. Lessaga, L.F. Eng, L.A. Sternberger, N.H. Sternberger, and H. Ulrich. 1988. An immunohistochemical study of the cerebellar cortex. *Acta Neuropathol.* 75: 474.

Sima, A.A.F., A.W. Clark, N.H. Sternberger, and L.A. Sternberger. 1986. Lewy body dementia without Alzheimer changes. *Can. J. Neurol. Sci.* 13: 440.

Sternberger, L.A. 1986. *Immunochemistry*, 3rd edition. Wiley, New York.

Sternberger, L.A. and N.H. Sternberger. 1983. Monoclonal antibodies distinguish phosphorylated and non-phosphorylated neurofilaments *in situ. Proc. Natl. Acad. Sci.* 80: 6126.

Sternberger, L.A., L.W. Harwell, and N.H. Sternberger. 1982. Neurotypy: Regional individuality in rat brain detected by immunocytochemistry with monoclonal antibodies. *Proc. Natl. Acad. Sci.* 79: 1326.

Sternberger, L.A., P.H. Hardy, J.J. Cuculis, and H.G. Meyer. 1970. The unlabeled antibody enzyme method of immunohistochemistry: Preparation and properties of soluble antigen-antibody complex (horseradish peroxidase-antihorseradish peroxidase) and its use in identification of spirochetes. *J. Histochem. Cytochem.* 18: 315.

Sternberger, L.A., J. Ulrich, L. Guth, C.P. Barrett, and N.H. Sternberger. 1989. Neurofilament processing in trauma and disease. In *Cellular and molecular aspects of neural development and regeneration* (ed. B. Huber et al.). Springer Verlag, Heidelberg. (In press.)

Sternberger, N.H. and L.A. Sternberger. 1987. Blood-brain barrier-antigen recognized by monoclonal antibody. *Proc. Natl. Acad. Sci.* 84: 8169.

9

Sternberger, N.H., L.A. Sternberger, and J. Ulrich. 1985. Aberrant neurofilament phosphorylation in Alzheimer disease. *Proc. Natl. Acad. Sci.* **82:** 4274.

Neurofilament Proteins and Neuroectodermal Brain Tumors

J.Q. Trojanowski

Department of Pathology and Laboratory Medicine (Neuropathology)
The University of Pennsylvania School of Medicine
Philadelphia, Pennsylvania 19104-6079

Medulloblastomas are common childhood central nervous system (CNS) tumors that appear to be similar but are biologically heterogeneous (Burger and Vogel 1982; Rorke et al. 1985; Rubinstein 1985). In fact, medulloblastomas appear to be similar to a number of other childhood CNS and peripheral nervous system (PNS) tumors of putative neuronal derivation, i.e., neuroblastomas, pineoblastomas, retinoblastomas, and so forth. Little is known about the cell biology of medulloblastomas, nor is there agreement on how to classify these and other poorly differentiated brain tumors. Although morphological comparisons with normal neural cells are the basis for traditional classification schemes, CNS precursors that differentiate into neurons and glia are not readily identified by their morphology alone. Molecular markers of neuronal or glial differentiation could rectify this, and monoclonal antibodies (MAbs) to intermediate filament (IF) proteins have been used to enumerate the cells present in different neoplasms (for reviews, see Virtanen et al. 1985; Lehto et al. 1986; Osborn and Weber 1986; and this volume). However, the cell types in medulloblastomas have been subject to detailed analysis only recently with anti-IF MAbs. Following earlier efforts to use anti-neurofilament (NF) MAbs to identify neuron-like tumor cells in a variety of CNS and PNS neoplasms (see, e.g., Trojanowski et al. 1982, 1984), we have characterized the IF proteins in medulloblastomas. This overview provides a summary of recent efforts to exploit anti-IF MAbs to identify cell types in medulloblastomas and to understand the extent to which the IFs of these tumors are deranged in transformed neuron-like cells. Emphasis is placed on NF proteins because NFs are the major IFs of neurons. Recent reviews of NF structure and biochemistry (Schlaepfer 1987; Matus 1988), as well as NF protein expression in CNS and PNS tumors (Trojanowski 1988), provide additional background on this subject.

11

Neurofilament Proteins and Medulloblastomas:
An Overview of Recent Work

In one of the earlier studies of NF proteins in medulloblastomas, the presence of NF-positive tumor cells was noted (Roessmann et al. 1983). Our studies with subunit-specific anti-NF MAbs produced by Lee and co-workers revealed the presence of the high (NF-H), middle (NF-M), and low (NF-L) molecular-weight NF subunits, as well as glial fibrillary acidic protein (GFAP) and vimentin filament protein in biopsies of medulloblastomas (Tremblay et al. 1985). GFAP was the most commonly expressed IF protein, and NF subunits were uncommon. However, it was not always possible to distinguish reactive cells from tumor cells in biopsies. Furthermore, proof that proliferating brain tumor cells express differentiated gene products, such as NF proteins, requires the examination of tumor cell lines. With the subsequent availability of additional MAbs to different NF subunits that distinguished NF-H and NF-M in different states of phosphorylation and the production of medulloblastoma cell lines, it was feasible to probe the cell types in medulloblastomas.

A human medulloblastoma cell line (D283 MED), isolated by Friedman et al. (1985), was examined using immunochemical and immunohistochemical methods, and it was shown that this cell line expressed all three NF subunits but no other IF proteins except vimentin (Trojanowski et al. 1987). However, more than 90% of the cells contained NF-H and NF-M immunoreactivity, but less than 10% contained NF-L immunoreactivity. These studies provided the first molecular evidence that medulloblastomas contain a population of neoplastic cells that are capable of rapid cell division and the expression of NF proteins, the IF proteins of mature, nondividing neurons. Curiously, GFAP-positive cells were present in the initial brain biopsy specimen of the tumor from whence the D283 MED cell line was derived but not in the cell line or subcutaneous xenografts of the cell line. The results obtained with the MAb to GFAP raised the possibility that GFAP-positive cells in biopsy specimens of medulloblastomas arise from non-neoplastic glial cells trapped within the tumor, rather than from neoplastic components of the tumor. When Friedman et al. (1988) established another medulloblastoma cell line (D341), it was possible to extend our observations to this cell line and provide a second example of a NF-positive and GFAP-negative medulloblastoma cell line (Friedman et al. 1988). Despite similarities between D283 and D341, the latter cell line differed from the former because it was devoid of any NF-L, and only a minority of the cells (5–25%) expressed NF-H and/or NF-M. The only other well-established medulloblastoma cell lines, i.e., TE-671 (McAllister et al. 1977) and DAOY (Jacobsen et al. 1985), were examined next, and they were found to lack GFAP and NF immunoreactivity (He et al. 1989). Thus, although the number of medulloblastoma cell lines available for examination is limited, it is evident that phenotypic heterogeneity exists among these four cell lines at the level of their IF proteins. He et al. (1989) also noted additional molecular differences among them. These studies provided evidence that at least two medulloblastoma cell lines rapidly divide and express NF proteins that are immunologically and biochemically similar to human NF proteins. The nature of the GFAP-positive cells in biopsy samples of medulloblastomas remains enigmatic, but they may well represent reactive astrocytes. Data on the NF proteins expressed by these four cell lines are summarized in Table 1.

Although these studies answered important questions about the IFs of medulloblastomas, they raised additional questions concerning NF and other neuronal cytoskeletal proteins in medulloblastomas, such as, Are the NF subunits expressed by medulloblastomas normal or abnormal? Do assembled NFs exist in these tumor cells, and what is their function? Are perturbations of NFs necessary for tumor progression? Are other neuronal cytoskeletal proteins, i.e., microtubule-associated proteins (MAPs), normal or abnormal in medulloblastomas? If the cytoskeleton links the plasma membrane to the nucleus and plays a role in determining cell shape, cell motility, and cell-cell interactions, does the neuronal cytoskeleton of tumor cells contribute to the molecular events that lead to tumor progression? Finally, what is the prognostic significance of the selective expression of normal versus abnormal NF proteins in some medulloblastomas (biopsy samples, cell lines)?

Neuronal Cytoskeletal Proteins and Medulloblastomas: Future Directions

Additional studies will need to address these questions, but some answers are suggested by the studies reviewed above, as well as by more recent studies of these cell lines (Kelsten et al. 1988; Trojanowski et al. 1989). For example, data on the NF proteins of the four medulloblastoma cell lines suggest that the

Table 1 Neuronal and Glial Cytoskeletal Proteins in Human Medulloblastoma Cell Lines

MAb	Subunit specificity[a]	Phosphorylation state of epitope[a]	Epitope domain[b]	Cell line results[c]			
				D283	D341	TE-671	DAOY
RMS12	NF-L only	P(ind)	C	+*	–	–	–
RMO3	NF-M only	P(ind)	P	+	+	–	–
HO14	NF-M only	P(+)	P	+*	+	–	–
RMO123	NF-M only	P(+)	P	+	+	–	–
RMO254	NF-M only	P(ind)	P	+	+	–	–
RMO281	NF-M only	P(+)	P	+*	+	–	–
TA50	NF-H+NF-M	P(+)	P	+*	+*	–	–
RMdO20	NF-M+NF-H	P(–)	P	+	+	–	–
HO57	NF-H only	P(+)	P	+	+	±	±
RMO24	NF-H only	P(+)	P	–	–	–	–
RMO217	NF-H only	P(+)	P	–	–	–	–
TA51	NF-H only	P(+)	P	+*	+*	±	±
RMO304	NF-H only	P(–)	P	–	–	–	–
T14	τ only	P(ind)	83–120	–	–	–	–
T49	τ only	P(ind)	n.a.	–	–	–	–
M5, M12	MAP$_2$ only	P(ind)	n.a.	–	–	–	–
2.2B10	GFAP only	P(ind)	n.a.	–	–	–	–

[a](P(+)) Diminished immunoreactivity after dephosphorylation; (P(–)) increased immunoreactivity after dephosphorylation; (P(ind)) no change after dephosphorylation.

[b](C) Core; (P) carboxy-terminal peripheral; (83–120) amino acids in τ within which the T14 epitope is located; (n.a.) not available.

[c](+) Positive; (–) negative; (±) equivocal. MAbs that immunostained cells of a given line were also used to immunoblot cell homogenates; (*) MAbs that yielded immunobands corresponding to normal human spinal cord NF subunits. HO57 and TA51 stained some cells in TE-671 and DAOY, but these MAbs and RMS12 failed to detect immunobands in cell homogenates. For information on the cell lines, see He et al. (1989). The MAbs are described elsewhere (Carden et al. 1985, 1987; Kosik et al. 1988; Lee and Andrews 1986; Lee et al. 1986a,b, 1987, 1988a,b; Schmidt et al. 1987; Trojanowski et al. 1989).

NF proteins in D283 and D341 are abnormal compared with their counterparts in normal developing or mature (see, e.g., Shaw and Weber 1982; Sternberger and Sternberger 1983; Lee and Andrews 1986; Trojanowski et al. 1986; Lee et al. 1987; Black and Lee 1988) and maldeveloped (Yachnis et al. 1988) neurons for the following reasons: (1) NF immunoreactivity in medulloblastomas is arranged in perinuclear aggregates that are not seen in normal neurons but may be seen in transformed cells (Lee et al. 1982; Trojanowski et al. 1982, 1984; Lee 1985); (2) the majority of D283 and D341 cells lack immunoreactive NF-L but express NF-M and NF-H; (3) electron microscopic studies reveal few IFs, or the IFs are collapsed into perinuclear bundles and lack NF side arms; and (4) the phosphoisoforms of NF-H and NF-M are not distributed in perikarya versus processes like those of normal neurons. Furthermore, preliminary studies indicate that these cell lines do not coexpress τ and other MAPs, e.g., MAP_2 (Trojanowski et al. 1989; Table 1), and variants of NF-H and NF-M that arise as a result of their differential phosphorylation (phosphoisoforms) change very little as a function of the cell cycle (Kelsten et al. 1988).

It should now be possible to determine whether neuronal cytoskeletal proteins in medulloblastomas (compared with normal mature or developing neurons) result from tumor-specific alterations and whether the diverse neuron-like cells in medulloblastomas arise from genetic or posttranslational aberrations in these tumors. This information should lead to a more detailed understanding of the cell biology of medulloblastomas, and it can be exploited to classify and treat CNS and PNS tumors in a more effective manner.

ACKNOWLEDGMENTS
We express appreciation to Dr. V.M.-Y. Lee for helpful collaboration. Ms. T. Schuck and Ms. C. Page contributed invaluably in all aspects of this work. Dr. V. LiVolsi of the Hospital of the University of Pennsylvania and Drs. R. Packer and L. Rorke of Childrens Hospital of Philadelphia contributed tissue for some of the studies described here. Drs. D. Bigner and H. Friedman made the four medulloblastoma cell lines available for collaboration and study. We thank Dr. W.M. Molenaar for her comments on this manuscript. Work discussed here was supported primarily by CA-36245 (a MERIT Award from the National Cancer Institute).

REFERENCES

Black, M.M. and V.M.-Y. Lee. 1988. Phosphorylation of neurofilament proteins in intact neurons: Demonstration of phosphorylation in cell bodies and axons. *J. Neurosci.* **8:** 3296.

Burger, P.C. and F.S. Vogel. 1982. *Surgical pathology of the nervous system and its coverings*, 2nd edition. Wiley, Baltimore.

Carden, M.J., W.W. Schlaepfer, and V.M.-Y. Lee. 1985. The structure, biochemical properties, and immunogenicity of neurofilament peripheral regions are determined by phosphorylation state. *J. Biol. Chem.* **260:** 9805.

Carden, M.J., J.Q. Trojanowski, W.W. Schlaepfer, and V.M.-Y. Lee. 1987. Two-stage expression of neurofilament polypeptides during rat neurogenesis with early establishment of adult phosphorylation patterns. *J. Neurosci.* **7:** 3489.

Friedman, H.S., P.C. Burger, S.H. Bigner, J.Q. Trojanowski, C.J. Wikstrand, E.C. Halperin, and D.D. Bigner. 1985. Establishment and characterization of the human medulloblastoma cell line and transplantable xenograft D283 MED. *J. Neuropathol. Exp. Neurol.* **44:** 592.

Friedman, H.S., P.C. Burger, S.H. Bigner, J.Q. Trojanowski, G.M. Brodeur, X. He, C.J. Wikstrand, J. Kurtzberg, M.E. Berens, E.C. Halperin, and D.D. Bigner. 1988. Phenotypic and genotypic analysis of a human medulloblastoma cell line and transplantable xenograft (D341 Med) demonstrating amplifications of c-*myc. Am. J. Pathol.* **130:** 472.

He, X., S. Skapek, C.J. Wikstrand, H.S. Friedman, J.Q. Trojanowski, J.T. Kemstead, H.B. Coakham, S.H. Bigner, and D.D. Bigner. 1989. Phenotypic analysis of four human medulloblastoma cell lines and transplantable xenografts. *J. Neuropathol. Exp. Neurol.* (in press).

Jacobsen, P.F., D.J. Jenkyn, and J.M. Papadimitriou. 1985. Establishment of a human medulloblastoma cell line and its heterotransplantation into nude mice. *J. Neuropathol. Exp. Neurol.* **44:** 472.

Kelsten, M., J.Q. Trojanowski, L. Lee, C. Clevenger, and D. Chianese. 1988. Neurofilament protein phospho-isoforms and the cell cycle in a human medulloblastoma cell line (D283 MED). *Cytometery* (suppl.) **2:** 66.

Kosik, K.S., L.D. Orrechio, L. Binder, J.Q. Trojanowski, V.M.-Y. Lee, and G. Lee. 1988. Epitopes that nearly span the tau molecule are shared with neurofibrillary tangles. *Neuron* (in press).

Lee, V.M.-Y. 1985. Neurofilament protein abnormalities in PC12 cells: Comparison with neurofilament proteins of normal cultured rat sympathetic neurons. *J. Neurosci.* **5:** 3039.

Lee, V.M.-Y. and P.W. Andrews. 1986. Differentiation of NTERA-2 clonal human embryonal carcinoma cells into neurons involves the induction of all three neurofilament proteins. *J. Neurosci.* **6:** 514.

Lee, V.M.-Y., M.J. Carden, and W.W. Schlaepfer. 1986a. Structural similarities and differences between neurofilament proteins from five different species as revealed using monoclonal antibodies. *J. Neurosci.* **6:** 2179.

Lee, V.M.-Y., M.J. Carden, and J.Q. Trojanowski. 1986b. Novel monoclonal antibodies provide evidence for the *in situ* existence of a non-phosphorylated form of the largest neurofilament subunit. *J. Neurosci.* **6:** 850.

Lee, V.M.-Y., J.Q. Trojanowski, and W.W. Schlaepfer. 1982. Induction of neurofilament triplet proteins in PC12 cells by NGF. *Brain Res.* **238:** 169.

Lee, V.M.-Y., M.J. Carden, W.W. Schlaepfer, and J.Q. Trojanowski. 1987. Monoclonal antibodies distinguish several differentially phosphorylated states of the two largest rat neurofilament subunits (NF-H and NF-M) and demonstrate their existence in the normal nervous system. *J. Neurosci.* **7:** 3474.

Lee, V.M.-Y., L. Otvos, M.L. Schmidt, and J.Q. Trojanowski. 1988a. Alzheimer's neurofibrillary tangles share immunological homologies with multiphosphorylation domains in the two large neurofilament proteins. *Proc. Natl. Acad. Sci.* **85:** 7384.

Lee, V.M.-Y., L. Otvos, M.J. Carden, M. Hollosi, B. Dietzschold, and R.A. Lazzarini. 1988b. Identification of the major multi-phosphorylation site in mammalian neurofilaments. *Proc. Natl. Acad. Sci.* **85:** 1998.

Lehto, V.-P., M. Miettinen, and I. Virtanen. 1986. Antibodies to intermediate filaments in surgical pathology. *Arch. Geschwulstforsch.* **56:** 283.

Matus, A. 1988. Neurofilament protein phosphorylation — Where, when and why. *Trends Neurochem. Sci.* **11:** 291.

McAllister, R.M., H. Isaacs, R. Rongey, M. Peer, W. Au, S.W. Soukup, and M.B. Gardner. 1977. Establishment of a human medulloblastoma cell line. *Int. J. Cancer* **20:** 206.

Osborn, M. and K. Weber. 1986. Intermediate filament proteins: A multigene family distinguishing major cell lineages. *Trends Biochem. Sci.* **11:** 469.

Roessmann, U., M.E. Velasco, P. Gambetti, and L. Autilio-Gambetti. 1983. Neuronal and astrocytic differentiation in human neuroepithelial neoplasms: An immunohistochemical study. *J. Neuropathol. Exp. Neurol.* **42:** 113.

Rorke, L.B., F.H. Gilles, F.L. Davis, and L.E. Becker. 1985. A revision of the World Health Organization classification of brain tumors for childhood brain tumors. *Cancer* **56:** 1869.

Rubinstein, L.J. 1985. A commentary on the proposed revision of the World Health Organization classification of brain tumors for childhood brain tumors. *Cancer* **56:** 1869.

Schlaepfer, W.W. 1987. Neurofilaments: Structure, metabolism and implications in disease. *J. Neuropathol. Exp. Neurol.* **46:** 117.

Schmidt, L.M., M.J. Carden, V.M.-Y. Lee, and J.Q. Trojanowski. 1987. Phosphorylated and non-phosphorylated neurofilament epitopes in the axonal swellings of patients with motor neuron disease and controls. *Lab. Invest.* **56:** 282.

Shaw, G. and K. Weber. 1982. Differential expression of neurofilament triplet proteins in brain development. *Nature* **298:** 277.

Sternberger, L.A. and N.H. Sternberger. 1983. Monoclonal antibodies distinguish phosphorylated and non-phosphorylated forms of neurofilaments *in situ. Proc. Natl. Acad. Sci.* **80:** 6126.

Tremblay, G.F., V.M.-Y. Lee, and J.Q. Trojanowski. 1985. Expression of vimentin, glial filament, and neurofilament proteins in primitive childhood brain tumors: A comparative immunoblot and immunoperoxidase study. *Acta Neuropathol.* **68:** 239.

Trojanowski, J.Q. 1988. Immunohistochemistry of neurofilament proteins and their diagnostic applications. In *Diagnostic immunohistochemistry* (ed. R.A. DeLellis), p. 237. Raven Press, New York.

Trojanowski, J.Q., V.M.-Y. Lee, and W.W. Schlaepfer. 1984. An immunohistochemical study of central and peripheral nervous system tumors with monoclonal antibodies against neurofilaments and glial filaments. *Hum. Pathol.* **15:** 248.

Trojanowski, J.Q., N. Walkenstein, and V.M.-Y. Lee. 1986. Expression of neurofilament subunits in neurons of the central and peripheral nervous system: An immunohistochemical study with monoclonal antibodies. *J. Neurosci.* **6:** 650.

Trojanowski, J.Q., H.S. Friedman, P.C. Burger, and D.D. Bigner. 1987. A rapidly dividing human medulloblastoma cell line (D283 MED) expresses all three neurofilament subunits. *Am. J. Pathol.* **126:** 358.

Trojanowski, J.Q., V. Lee, N. Pillsbury, and S. Lee. 1982. Neuronal origin of human esthesioneuroblastoma demonstrated with antineurofilament monoclonal antibodies. *N. Engl. J. Med.* **307:** 159.

Trojanowski, J.Q., T. Schuck, M.L. Schmidt, and V.M.-Y. Lee. 1989. The distribution of tau in the normal human nervous system. *J. Histochem. Cytochem.* (in press).

Virtanen, I., M. Miettinin, L.-P. Lehto, A.-L. Karminiemi, and R. Paasivuo. 1985. Diagnostic application of monoclonal antibodies to intermediate filaments. *Ann. N.Y. Acad. Sci.* **455:** 635.

Yachnis, T., J.Q. Trojanowski, M. Memmo, and W.W. Schlaepfer. 1988. Expression of neurofilament proteins in the hypertrophic granule cells of Lhermitte Duclos disease: An explanation for the mass effect and the myelination of parallel fibers in the disease state. *J. Neuropathol. Exp. Neurol.* **47:** 206.

The 58-kD Neuronal Intermediate Filament, Peripherin: Chemistry, Development, and Localization

M.L. Shelanski, C.M. Troy, C.H. Rhodes,[1]
J. Aletta, R.K.H. Liem, and L.A. Greene

Department of Pathology and Center for Neurobiology and Behavior
College of Physicians & Surgeons
Columbia University, New York, New York 10032
[1]Department of Pathology, University of Pennsylvania
Philadelphia, Pennsylvania 19104

Recently, it has become clear that in addition to the neurofilament (NF), mature mammalian neurons may contain a second neuron-specific intermediate filament (IF). This protein, named peripherin by Portier and her co-workers, was initially described in neuroblastoma and PC12 cells (Portier et al. 1983/1984b) and subsequently in a variety of peripheral neurons (Portier et al. 1983/1984a; Parysek and Goldman 1987). In addition to the peripheral nervous system (PNS), peripherin appears to be present in subsets of adult and embryonic mammalian central neurons (Leonard et al. 1988; Parysek and Goldman 1988; Parysek et al. 1988). The protein has an apparent molecular weight of 58,000 on SDS-polyacrylamide gels. A nerve growth factor (NGF)-regulated mRNA identified in PC12 cells by differential screening of cDNA libraries (Leonard et al. 1987) has now been established to encode peripherin (Aletta et al. 1988; Leonard et al. 1988). Analysis of the deduced amino acidic sequence of peripherin (Leonard et al. 1988) has shown it to be a member of the IF multigene, which is distinct from its other members.

Localization studies using in situ hybridization show message to be present in a variety of central neurons, including those in the oculomotor, trochlear, trigeminal (motor), abducens, facial, vagal, and hypoglossal nuclei. Message is also present in the motor neurons of the ventral horn of the spinal cord. No localization has been seen to nonneuronal cells in either the central nervous system (CNS) or the PNS.

We have prepared three different antibodies against the peripherin molecule. The first was raised in rabbits against the purified filament protein from PC12 cells. The second is also a rabbit polyclonal raised against a synthetic 19-mer near the carboxy-terminal region of the protein predicted from the cDNA sequence of clone-73 mRNA (Leonard et al. 1988). The third is a monoclonal antibody directed to a region near the amino terminus of the protein. All of these antibodies have been tested in immunoblots and by immunostaining. The studies presented here rely solely on the antisynthetic peptide antibody that has given the strongest immunostaining of the three. This antibody recognizes the PC12 58-kD IF, staining in a clearly filamentous pattern and blotting on two-dimensional immunoblots. Partial sequence analysis of the PC12 protein shows a complete homology with the clone-73 sequence.

Peripherin separates into five distinct isoforms on two-dimensional gel electrophoresis. Three of these isoforms are phosphorylated when PC12 cells are labeled with [^{32}P] ortho-phosphate, and this phosphorylation is markedly stimulated by NGF and moderately stimulated by activators of protein kinases A and C or depolarizing levels of K^+. Over 90% of total peripherin in the PC12 cells is in the assembled form. It is unclear whether the small amount that is soluble represents protomers or degradation product. Similar isoforms are seen in the sciatic nerve of the rat.

We have begun a comparison of the development of peripherin and neurofilaments in the mouse embryo from E8 to E18. A limited number of nerve fibers are stained with peripherin at E9, although cellular staining is lacking with either anti-NF or anti-peripherin. At E10, peripherin is present in the cell bodies of dorsal root ganglions (DRGs) and in many nerve fibers. NF staining is also present but is much stronger in processes than in cell bodies. At E11, the anterior horn cells and anterior roots show clear peripherin staining, whereas they are negative for NF-M (middle). Our preliminary data show strong peripherin staining in DRG, sympathetic ganglion, nodose ganglion, gasserian ganglion, and peripheral nerves at E12. Strong peripherin staining is present in the ascending tracts of the dorsal columns. Weaker peripherin staining is present in a group of unidentified cells in the midbrain. No peripherin staining was seen in higher brain structures or the retina. Peripherin and NF proteins are both present in DRGs and superior cervical ganglions with approximately the same distribution at E17, whereas peripherin remains the major filament present in the perikarya of anterior horn cells. The same general distribution of peripherin in other ganglia is found at E17 as was seen at E12. Adult distributions closely parallel those at E17.

We have used the anti-peripherin antibody to stain a variety of tumors from the CNS. The best results have been obtained on unfixed frozen sections. Results on deparaffinized slides have been equivocal, although the reasons for this are unclear. In these studies, no staining has been seen in the cells of a variety of astrocytomas ranging in type from highly differentiated to anaplastic. In some cases, a nonspecific background staining was seen. Nerve cell processes entrapped in the tumor were peripherin-positive, on occasion. No cellular staining was seen in a craniopharyngioma, a pituitary adenoma, a meningioma, or a schwannoma. Cultures of the U251 human astrocytoma line were also negative. Positive staining was seen in several medulloblastomas and in two gangliogliomas. The cells were strongly positive for peripherin in one medulloblastoma while expressing little, if any, neurofilament staining. Cultures of human neuroblastoma were also peripherin-positive.

In summary, peripherin is a useful marker for neurons and their processes, especially where they are derived from the PNS and brain-stem nuclei. In many cases, peripherin and the neurofilament proteins are present in the same cell and often have the same distribution within the cell. In other cases, their respective localizations and configurations appear to diverge, suggesting that they may subserve discrete functions. Preliminary data suggest that the antibody to peripherin might be of utility in the diagnosis of tumors that contain elements of neuronal lineage.

REFERENCES

Aletta, J.M., R. Angeletti, R.K.H. Liem, C. Purcell, M.L. Shelanski, and L.A. Green. 1988. Relationship between the nerve growth factor-regulated clone 73 gene product and the 58-kilodalton neuronal intermediate filament protein (peripherin). *J. Neurochem.* **51**:1317.

Leonard, D.G.B., E.G. Ziff, and L.A. Greene. 1987. Identification and characterization of mRNAs regulated by nerve growth factor in PC12 cells. *Mol. Cell. Biol.* **7**: 3156.

Leonard, D.G.B., J.D. Gorham, P. Cole, L.A. Greene, and E.G. Ziff. 1988. A nerve growth factor-regulated messenger RNA encodes a new intermediate filament protein. *J. Cell. Biol.* **106**: 181.

Parysek, L.M. and R.D. Goldman. 1987. Characterization of intermediate filaments in PC12 cells. *J. Neurosci.* **7**: 781.

————. 1988. Distribution of a novel 57 kDa intermediate filament (IF) protein in the nervous system. *J. Neurosci.* **8:** 555.

Parysek, L.M., R.L. Chisholm, C.A. Ley, and R.D. Goldman. 1988. A type III intermediate filament gene is expressed in mature neurons. *Neuron* **1:** 395.

Portier, M.-M., B. de Néchaud, and F. Gros. 1983/1984a. Peripherin, a new member of the intermediate filament protein family. *Dev. Neurosci.* **6:** 335.

Portier, M.-M., P. Brachet, B. Croizat, and F. Gros. 1983/1984b. Regulation of peripherin in mouse neuroblastoma and rat PC12 pheochromocytoma cell lines. *Dev. Neurosci.* **6:** 215.

Neuroendocrine and Nerve Sheath Neoplasms

V.E. Gould[1] and D. Jansson[1,2]

[1]Department of Pathology, Rush Medical College
Chicago, Illinois 60612

[2]Department of Pathology, Swedish University of
Agricultural Sciences, S-750 07 Uppsala, Sweden

Neuroendocrine (NE) differentiation is of fundamental evolutionary significance. Molecules such as insulin, bombesin, and cholecystokinin have been identified through all vertebrates, and similar molecules are also present in arthropods, mollusks, protozoa, fungi, and even bacteria, where they can be demonstrated with antibodies to their mammalian counterparts, thus attesting to a remarkable degree of molecular conservation (Falkmer et al. 1984).

NE cells comprise a heterogeneous family forming the dispersed neuroendocrine system (DNS). As currently understood, the DNS includes central and peripheral neurons, adrenal medullae and paraganglia, traditional endocrine glands such as the hypophysis, less well-defined cellular aggregates such as pancreatic islets and pulmonary neuro-epithelial bodies (NEBs), parafollicular thyroid cells, and a large number of widely distributed cells demonstrable in the mucosa of the gastrointestinal, bronchopulmonary, and urogenital tracts, the skin, and so forth (Gould et al. 1985).

Structurally, the common denominator of NE cells is the presence of 30–60-nm-diameter "empty" appearing vesicles and larger, 80–400-nm-diameter neurosecretory granules with a variably dense core. Their functional commonality rests on their ability to produce certain amino acids, amines, and peptides that, in different sites, can variably act as neurotransmitters, paracrine modulators, and/or true hormones.

NE differentiation is not restricted to cells derived from any given embryonal germ layer or structure. The intermediate filament (IF) complement of NE cells reflects that heterogeneity: Neurons and paraganglia express neurofilament protein (NFP), whereas epithelial NE cells express cytokeratin polypeptides of simple epithelial type. Furthermore, certain

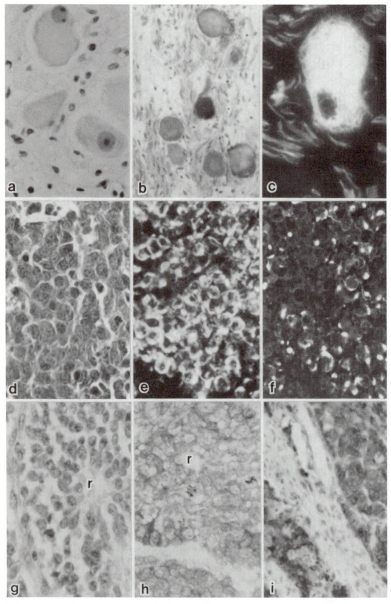

Figure 1 (*See facing page for legend.*)

24

cells such as melanocytes may express NE differentiation, whereas their IF complement is of mesenchymal type, e.g., exclusively vimentin.

On the basis of their cytoskeletal characteristics, NE neoplasms may be divided into three groups: (1) purely or predominantly neural, (2) purely or predominantly epithelial, and (3) miscellaneous, in which vimentin is the exclusive or predominant IF protein.

Neural NE Neoplasms

Ganglioneuromas are benign neoplasms occurring mostly in young adults; frequent sites are the posterior mediastinum and the retroperitoneal space. They consist of variable numbers of mature ganglion cells, e.g., neurons, and a network of dendritic processes (Fig. 1a–c). Pheochromocytomas develop in the adrenal medulla; they display solid cellular aggregates separated by abundant fibrovascular stroma. Paragangliomas are similar to pheochromocytomas but arise from extraadrenal paraganglia in the posterior mediastinum, retroperitoneum, and some viscera. Neuroblastomas are the highly malignant counterparts of pheochromocytomas. They develop in the adrenal medulla and paraganglia of infants and children. Neural tumors also develop in the mucosa of the upper nasal passages and paranasal sinuses; these include esthesioneuroepitheliomas and neuroblastomas. With the exception of pheochromocytomas, neural NE tumors seldom present with hormonal manifestations.

Ultrastructurally, all of these tumors show variable complements of neurosecretory granules besides the characteristic

Figure 1 (*a–c*) Ganglioneuroma of posterior mediastinum. (*a*) Numerous ganglion cells, HE; (*b*) staining with antibody to VIP (vasoactive intestinal polypeptide) is noted in cell bodies and processes (ABC method on paraffin section); (*c*) staining with antibody to 68-kD subunit of NFP also involves cell body and processes; note the unstained nucleus (immunofluorescence on frozen section). (*d–f*) Neuroendocrine skin carcinoma. (*d*) Neoplastic infiltrate in the dermis, HE; (*e*) staining with pan-cytokeratin antibody (immunofluorescence on frozen section); (*f*) staining with antibody cocktail, including the three NFP subunits (immunofluorescence on frozen section). (*g–i*) Primitive neuroectodermal tumor of soft tissue (lower limb). (*g*) Rosette-like structure (r) amid irregular aggregate of small cells, HE; (*h*) diffuse and uniform vimentin staining; a rosette (r) (ABC method on frozen section); (*i*) different area of the same tumor showing intense staining with antibody cocktail, including the three NFP subunits (ABC method on frozen section).

25

small vesicles. Immunohistochemically, neuron-specific enolase (NSE), synaptophysin, and chromogranins, as well as serotonin and neuropeptides, may be shown with variable frequency in literally all of these tumors, regardless of the presence or absence of clinical hormonal activity.

Irrespective of type, clinical manifestations, or hormonal activity, these tumors express variable admixtures of the three NFP subunits, apparently unassociated with desmoplakins (Osborn et al. 1986). A subset of olfactory neural tumors coexpress NFP with cytokeratins (Taxy et al. 1986); recently, the PC12 rat pheochromocytoma cell line has been shown to coexpress NFP and cytokeratin polypeptides and desmoplakins (Franke et al. 1986). Some neural NE tumors may include a subpopulation of Schwann-like cells that express vimentin and may occasionally produce melanin.

Epithelial NE Neoplasms

These are the most frequent and widely distributed NE neoplasms. Carcinoids are classic examples of the benign or low-grade malignant epithelial NE tumors. They arise typically in the gastrointestinal tract or bronchi. They consist of solid cell clusters and ribbons with a rich fibrovascular stroma; pleomorphism is minimal. Other benign epithelial NE tumors include adenomas of the anterior hypophysis, parathyroid glands, and pancreatic islets. Malignant epithelial NE tumors are generically termed NE carcinomas. They arise in the bronchi, gastrointestinal tract, skin (Fig. 1d–f), uterine cervix, thymus, pancreas, and miscellaneous sites; medullary thyroid carcinomas also belong to this group. Epithelial NE tumors may present with hormonal syndromes related to overproduction of eutopic or "ectopic" hormones. Most cases do not present with clinical syndromes, yet NE substances may be detected and measured in the serum.

Electron microscopy indicates that heterogeneous neurosecretory granules are the common denominator of epithelial NE tumors; they are abundant in carcinoids but may be exceedingly rare in the less differentiated NE carcinomas. Regardless of hormonal activity, NSE, chromogranin, synaptophysin, serotonin, and neuropeptides can be shown immunocytochemically with variable frequency and in different combinations.

Epithelial NE tumors express cytokeratin polypeptides of simple epithelial type (nos. 8, 18, and 19) and desmoplakins

26

(Blobel et al. 1985). Subsets of bronchial carcinoids, islet cell and parathyroid adenomas, NE skin carcinomas, and most medullary thyroid carcinomas, among others, coexpress cytokeratins—NFP and desmoplakins (Gould et al. 1985). Cytokeratin-vimentin coexpression is often detected in diverse types of NE carcinoma cells growing in effusions. In tissue, vimentin is noted in rare medullary thyroid carcinomas (Dockhorn-Dworniczak et al. 1987), as well as in Schwann-like cell subpopulations present in some carcinoids and medullary thyroid carcinomas. These latter cells may also produce melanin.

Miscellaneous NE Neoplasms

Melanocytes are found in the skin and some mucosal and meningeal surfaces; they are neural crest derivatives, putative members of the DNS, and express vimentin. Normal melanocytes have structural and functional features reminiscent of their neural ancestry. By immunocytochemistry, benign melanocytic tumors (e.g., nevi) can be readily shown to express NE markers such as NSE, serotonin, and some neuropeptides. Whereas only rare malignant melanomas present clinical hormonal syndromes, NE markers such as NSE, serotonin, calcitonin, gastrin, ACTH, enkephalins, and somatostatin have been noted in a number of them (Gould et al. 1985). Despite this wide spectrum of functional capabilities, malignant melanomas remain exclusive vimentin producers. This feature is retained during in vitro culture and in nude mice xenografts.

Medulloblastomas are infancy and childhood tumors occurring anywhere in the central nervous system (CNS) but mostly in the cerebellum; they are said to derive from "primitive neural cells." Microscopically, they may recapitulate aspects of the CNS development. Ultrastructurally, neural features are noted; immunocytochemically, some medulloblastomas stain for NSE and synaptophysin. Their IF complement is variable: Vimentin alone or coexpressed with glial fibrillar protein (GFP) and NFP may be demonstrated (Gould et al. 1986a). Primitive neuroectodermal tumors (PNETs) comprise a recently defined group of tumors arising in diverse sites including bone and soft tissues (Fig. 1g–i); they share many features with medulloblastomas, which indeed may be part of the group (Rorke 1983). PNETs may express NE markers including NSE and synaptophysin, whereas their IF complement is complex: Vimentin alone or coexpressed with NFP, GFP, and cytokeratins may be shown.

Nerve Sheath Neoplasms

Normal nerve sheath cells express vimentin; a few may coexpress GFP, although this may vary among species. Benign nerve sheath tumors include classic schwannomas and neurofibromas and variants thereof, granular cell tumors, and nerve sheath myxomas. All of these tumors have malignant counterparts. This heterogeneous group of tumors express vimentin; notably, a subset of benign schwannomas and neurofibromas have been shown to coexpress GFP by immunohistochemistry (Gould et al. 1986b).

EPILOG

NE cells comprising the DNS are diverse and widely distributed; they include elements derived from different embryonal structures that express a common NE program but whose IF complement may be neural, epithelial, or mesenchymal. NE neoplasms are frequent and clinically and morphologically heterogeneous. The variability of the IF complement of normal NE cells is not only retained but exaggerated in the corresponding neoplasms.

Thus, neural NE neoplasms retain the NFP expression of normal neural cells but are capable of coexpressing cytokeratin polypeptides at least in vitro. Similarly, epithelial NE tumors retain the simple epithelium-type cytokeratin polypeptides expressed by their ancestors, but subsets of both benign and malignant variants may coexpress NFP and rarely vimentin. Miscellaneous NE tumors mimicking embryonal CNS development retain the expression of vimentin but may coexpress GFP and NFP, whereas vimentin predominates in PNETs of soft tissue or bone; but the presumably aberrant coexpression of NFP, GFP, and cytokeratins may be added. Evidently, the diagnostic application of IF antibodies to NE tumors does not lend itself to facile simplifications for NE neoplasms cut across diverse lines of differentiation, and their IF complement may differ considerably from that of nonneoplastic cells of the same sites. Similarly, in nerve sheath neoplasms, the expression of vimentin parallels that of normal nerve sheath cells; however, a subset of tumors at the benign end of the spectrum may coexpress GFP.

These and other findings also point out that tumor classifications based on traditional notions of "histogenesis" may not be tenable in view of the complexity of differentiation, the plasticity, and the relative "infidelity" of expression exhibited by transformed populations. Nevertheless, IF antibodies are extremely useful as investigative and diagnostic tools in the study of NE neoplasms, especially when applied in concert with conventional clinicopathologic data, other appropriate immunoprobes, and adjunct biochemical techniques.

REFERENCES

Blobel, G.A., V.E. Gould, R. Moll, I. Lee, M. Huszar, B. Geiger, and W.W. Franke. 1985. Coexpression of neuroendocrine markers and epithelial cytoskeletal proteins in bronchopulmonary neuroendocrine neoplasms. *Lab. Invest.* **52:** 39.

Dockhorn-Dworniczak, B., W.W. Franke, S. Schroeder, B. Czernobilsky, V.E. Gould, and W. Boecker. 1987. Patterns of expression of cytoskeletal proteins in human thyroid gland and thyroid carcinomas. *Differentiation* **35:** 53.

Falkmer, S., R. Hakanson, and F. Sundler, eds. 1984. *Evolution and tumor pathology of the neuroendocrine system.* Elsevier, Amsterdam.

Franke, W.W., C. Grund, and T. Achstaetter. 1986. Coexpression of cytokeratins and neurofilament proteins in a permanent cell line: Cultured rat PC12 cells combine neuronal and epithelial features. *J. Cell Biol.* **103:** 1933.

Gould, V.E., R. Moll, I. Moll, I. Lee, and W.W. Franke. 1985. Neuroendocrine (Merkel) cells of the skin: Hyperplasias, dysplasias, and neoplasms. *Lab. Invest.* **52:** 334.

Gould, V.E., I. Lee, B. Wiedenmann, R. Moll, G. Chejfec, and W.W. Franke. 1986a. Synaptophysin: A novel marker for neurons, certain neuroendocrine cells and their neoplasms. *Hum. Pathol.* **17:** 979.

Gould, V.E., R. Moll, I. Moll, I. Lee, K. Schwechheimer, and W.W. Franke. 1986b. The intermediate filament complement of the spectrum of nerve sheath neoplasms. *Lab. Invest.* **55:** 463.

Osborn, M., T. Dirk, H. Kaeser, K. Weber, and M. Altmannsberger. 1986. Immunohistochemical localization of neurofilaments and neuron-specific enolase in 29 cases of neuroblastoma. *Am. J. Pathol.* **122:** 433.

Rorke, L.B. 1983. The cerebellar neuroblastoma and its relationship to primitive neuroectodermal tumors. *J. Neuropathol. Exp. Neurol.* **42:** 1.

Taxy, J.B., N.K. Bharani, S.E. Mills, H.F. Frierson, and V.E. Gould. 1986. The spectrum of olfactory neural tumors. *Am. J. Surg. Pathol.* **10:** 687.

Recent Advances in the Molecular Biology of Lung Cancer Having Clinical Implications

A.F. Gazdar and J.D. Minna

NCI-Navy Medical Oncology Branch, National Cancer Institute
and Naval Hospital, Bethesda, Maryland 20814

Lung cancer is the most common cause of cancer deaths in North America. Unfortunately, therapeutic advances have been of modest benefit, and nearly 90% of patients will eventually succumb from their disease (Minna et al. 1985). In an effort to develop more rational approaches to therapy, we have invested more than a decade of clinico-laboratory effort in studying the pathobiology of lung cancer. In this paper, we review recent advances in this field having potential clinical implications. It is important to realize that this summary represents the efforts of several investigators in our laboratory and elsewhere.

Four areas of molecular biology will be discussed. (1) Differentiation genes may be expressed in an appropriate or an inappropriate setting; they also may play a role in drug resistance. (2) Peptides and other growth factors may be secreted by tumor cells (autocrine secretion); in addition, expression of receptors may regulate growth and expression of the malignant phenotype. (3) Oncogenes may play a role in the pathogenesis of malignancy, as well as in tumor progression. Abnormalities of copy number (amplification), overexpression, and point mutations have been described in lung cancers. (4) Deletions of genes expressed in many normal cells may play a role in the appearance or maintenance of the malignant state. These "anti-oncogenes" represent one of the newest and most intriguing areas of study.

On clinical grounds, lung cancers may be divided into two broad subgroups: small-cell lung cancer (SCLC) and non-SCLC (NSCLC). SCLC tumors are relatively sensitive to cytotoxic therapies initially, but later relapse, at which time they are resistant to most agents (multidrug resistance). In contrast, most NSCLC tumors demonstrate multidrug resistance at the time of diagnosis. There are also important biological reasons for this basic subdivision. SCLC and the related bronchial carcinoid are typical neuroendocrine (NE) tumors (Gazdar et al. 1988). The primary function of NE cells is the production of specific peptide and amine products. In addition to these specific products, NE cells share many common properties. Included among these general markers is the presence of cytoplasmic dense-core cytoplasmic granules, the storage site of the specific products. The granules contain chromogranin A, a matrix protein, and NE cells express L-dopa decarboxylase, an enzyme essential for amine production. We and others have found that about 12% of NSCLC tumors and cell lines express multiple NE markers (Gazdar et al. 1988). Surprisingly, in vitro drug sensitivity testing of these NSCLC-NE tumors demonstrated that they were highly sensitive to all cytotoxic agents tested, similar in range to SCLC. We are currently testing whether NE differentiation in NSCLC is accompanied by an improved thereapeutic response.

As mentioned previously, multidrug resistance, occurring either de novo or post-therapy, is a common occurrence in all types of lung cancers. Although there are several possible mechanisms by which such multidrug resistance can occur, the best studied form is expression of a membrane P-glycoprotein associated with drug efflux (Pastan and Gottesman 1987), which is coded by the *MDR1* gene. S.-L. Lai (unpubl.) and others have studied expression of the *MDR1* gene in normal and malignant lung tissues and in lung cancer cell lines. With the exception of drug-sensitive NSCLC-NE and drug-resistant carcinoid tumors, expression of *MDR1* was low in all forms of lung cancer and did not correlate with in vitro sensitivity or with clinical response. We conclude that mechanisms other than *MDR1* expression are responsible for multidrug resistance in lung cancer. Unless verapamil and other calcium channel blockers reverse drug resistance by mechanisms other than affecting drug efflux, our data suggest that they will be ineffective in lung cancer.

For in vitro growth, cells require amino acids, glucose, a source for lipids, vitamins, salts, and buffers, which are provided by the basal growth medium. In addition, they require insulin- and transferrin-like growth factors, trace metals, steroid hormones, and other specific factors, which are usually provided by serum supplementation. However, if the precise requirements of a cell type are known, they may be supplied by a serum-free fully defined medium. Finally, tumor cells may make some of the factors that stimulate their own growth (autocrine secretion). F. Cuttitta, R. Natale, and J. Mulshine have identified many of these factors (Nakanishi et al. 1988), and they include insulin- and transferrin-like factors. SCLC tumors secrete many peptide products characteristic of NE cells. These include gastrin-releasing factor (GRP), a potent regulatory peptide. GRP is a well-documented autocrine factor. SCLC cells have specific GRP receptors, and their growth is stimulated in vitro and in xenografts by GRP. Of major interest is a monoclonal antibody to GRP, which inhibits the growth of SCLC. These observations have resulted in a clinical trial that tests the effects of anti-GRP antibody in relapsed SCLC patients.

The *myc* family is the group of proto-oncogenes most studied in lung cancer (Birrer and Minna 1988). All three members of the family, c-*myc*, N-*myc*, and L-*myc*, are expressed in normal lung. Although amplification of *myc* genes is seldom found in tumors and cell lines established from previously untreated SCLC patients, these genes are frequently amplified and over-expressed in tumors and cell lines from patients treated previously. B. Johnson has found that amplification of c-*myc* may be associated with shortened patient survival (Johnson et al. 1987). Amplification of c-*myc* is frequently associated with tumor progression of the variant subtype of SCLC (Johnson et al. 1987). This subtype, associated with poor clinical response, is characterized by large-cell morphology, rapid in vitro growth, and radioresistance (Gazdar et al. 1985).

Other oncogene abnormalities associated with lung cancer include point mutations of the *ras* family, especially in NSCLC, overexpression of P53 and c-*raf*-1, and amplification of c-*myb* (Birrer and Minna 1988).

A recent finding by J. Schutte (unpubl.) is of particular interest. He found c-*jun* in lung tissues and in many lung cancers and cell lines. Because *jun* is a transcriptional activator, affecting the transcription of several genes, overexpression of *jun* may regulate expression of the many specific cellular products associated with SCLC.

Although J. Whang-Peng et al. (1982) noted a specific chromosomal abnormality associated with SCLC in 1980, an interstitial deletion, 3p(14-23), her findings initially were controversial. However, using restriction-fragment-length polymorphism probes, her findings have been confirmed and extended by several laboratories (Johnson et al. 1988). Recently, W.

Harbour and F. Kaye have found frequent abnormalities of the retinoblastoma (*Rb*) gene in SCLC tumors and lines (Harbour et al. 1988). These findings strongly suggest that loss of genetic material (anti-oncogenes) on chromosomes 3 and 13 (and perhaps on other chromosomes) may play a role in the pathogenesis of SCLC. The exact incidence of these abnormalities in other forms of lung cancer is currently being studied.

Studies of biology and molecular genetics have greatly increased our knowledge of lung cancer. They form a sound basis for developing newer modalities for lung cancer diagnosis, staging, and therapy.

REFERENCES

Birrer, M.J. and J.D. Minna. 1988. Molecular genetics of lung cancer. *Semin. Oncol.* **15:** 226.

Gazdar, A.F., D.N. Carney, M.M. Nau, and J.D. Minna. 1985. Characterization of variant subclasses of cell lines derived from small cell lung cancer having distinctive biochemical, morphological and growth properties. *Cancer Res.* **45:** 2924.

Gazdar, A.F., L. Helman, M.A. Israel, E.K. Russell, I. Linnoila, J. Mulshine, H. Schuller, and J.G. Park. 1988. Expression of neuroendocrine cell markers L-dopa decarboxylase, chromogranin A, and dense core granules in human tumors of endocrine and non-endocrine origin. *Cancer Res.* **48:** 4078.

Harbour, J.W., S.L. Lai, J. Whang-Peng, A.F. Gazdar, J.D. Minna, and F.J. Kaye. 1988. Abnormalities in structure and expression of the human retinoblastoma gene in small cell lung cancer. *Science* **241:** 353.

Johnson, B.E., A.Y. Sakaguchi, A.F. Gazdar, J.D. Minna, D. Burch, A. Marshall, and S.L. Naylor. 1988. Restriction fragment length polymorphism studies show consistent loss of chromosome 3p alleles in small cell lung cancer patients' tumors. *J. Clin. Invest.* **82:** 502.

Johnson, B.E., D.C. Ihde, R.W. Makuch, A.F. Gazdar, D.N. Carney, H. Oie, E. Russell, M.M. Nau, and J.D. Minna. 1987. *myc* family oncogene amplification in tumor cell lines established from small cell lung cancer patients and its relationship to clinical status and course. *J. Clin. Invest.* **79:** 1629.

Minna, J.D., G.A. Higgins, and E.J. Glatstein. 1985. Cancer of the lung. In *Cancer: Principles and practice of oncology* (ed. V.T. DeVita et al.), p. 507. J.B. Lippincott, Philadelphia.

Nakanishi, Y., J.L. Mulshine, P.G. Kasprzyk, R.B. Natale, R. Maneckjee, I. Avis, A.M. Treston, A.F. Gazdar, J.D. Minna, and F. Cuttitta. 1988. Insulin-like growth factor-1 can mediate autocrine proliferation of human small cell lung cancer cell lines. *J. Clin. Invest.* **82:** 354.

Pastan, I. and M.M. Gottesman. 1987. Multiple drug resistance in human cancer. *N. Engl. J. Med.* **316:** 1388.

Whang-Peng, J., C.S. Kao-Shan, E.C. Lee, P.A. Bunn, D.C. Carney, A.F. Gazdar, and J.D. Minna. 1982. A specific chromosomal defect associated with human small cell lung cancer. *Science* **215:** 181.

Distinction of Small Round Cell Tumors of Children with Special Emphasis on Neuroblastoma and Rhabdomyosarcomas

M. Altmannsberger,[1] F. Wagner,[1] and M. Osborn[2]

[1]Department of Pathology, University of Giessen
Giessen, Federal Republic of Germany

[2]Max-Planck Institute for Biophysical Chemistry
Göttingen, Federal Republic of Germany

Differential diagnosis of small round cell tumors in childhood is very difficult. This group of tumors includes neuroblastoma, malignant lymphomas, Ewing's sarcoma, nephroblastoma, and rhabdomyosarcoma. To distinguish between the different entities, special methods such as electron microscopy and immunohistochemistry are usually employed. Even then, this group of tumors presents a special challenge, because the differential diagnosis is of importance for the subsequent clinical treatment. However, as is clear from Table 1, intermediate filament (IF) typing provides a relatively easy way to divide these tumors into subgroups. In this paper, we focus on neuroblastoma, rhabdomyosarcoma, nephroblastoma, and malignant lymphoma.

Neuroblastoma
Neuroblastomas are the most common solid tumors of infancy and childhood, excluding tumors of the central nervous system. When tested with antibodies against different neurofilaments, neurofilaments are expressed in all cases (Mukai et al. 1986; Osborn et al. 1986b). The staining pattern is heterogeneous, i.e., in undifferentiated neuroblastomas (Hughes grade III), areas with tumor cells positive for antibodies against the three neurofilament (NF) polypeptides alternate with areas negative for all antibodies (Fig. 1). It is also very interesting that there is no essential difference between the staining pattern of N52

Table 1 IF Protein Expression in Rhabdomyosarcoma, Neuroblastoma, Nephroblastoma, and Non-Hodgkin Lymphoma

Rhabdomyosarcoma	Desmin-positive; most cases coexpress desmin and vimentin;[a] titin-positive in well-differentiated tumors
Neuroblastoma	Neurofilament-triplet-positive; N52 and NE14 staining; Schwann cells express GFAP; further subdivision possible by cytogenetic studies
Nephroblastoma	Blastema: (a) Coexpression of keratin and vimentin (b) Only vimentin Tubules: Keratin-positive Stroma: Varying expression of vimentin, neurofilaments, and desmin
Non-Hodgkin lymphoma	Heterogeneous expression of vimentin; fibroblastic reticulum cells keratin-positive

[a]Coindre et al. (1988) have claimed keratin coexpression in 5% of their rhabdomyosarcoma cases.

and NE14 (Shaw et al. 1986). N52 is an antibody against NF-H (high), which detects a phosphorylation-independent epitope, whereas NE14 only reacts with phosphorylated epitopes. Well-differentiated neuroblastomas (grade II) and ganglioneuroblastomas (grade I) express the NF triple homogeneously. Unfortunately, the determination of NFs does not allow for the separation of prognostically good and bad cases and the distinction between classic neuroblastomas and so-called primitive neuroectodemal tumors (PNETs). This is possible through cytogenetic studies, as well as by antibodies directed against enzymes specific for sympathetic and parasympathetic cells (Thiele et al. 1987; Christiansen and Lampert 1988). Other types of IF proteins in neuroblastomas are only rarely expressed, e.g., vimentin and glial fibrillary acidic protein (GFAP) in spindle cells with Schwann cell differentiation (Gould et al. 1986).

Rhabdomyosarcomas

The most common soft tissue tumor in childhood is rhabdomyosarcoma. The embryonal and alveolar subtypes can be subdivided. In a previous study using mainly ethanol-fixed

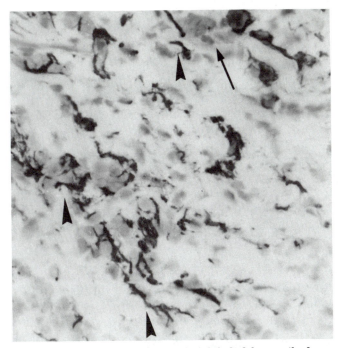

Figure 1 Neuroblastoma (Hughes III) labeled by antibody against NF-H (N52). The staining is heterogeneous. Positive areas are indicated by arrowheads; negative tumor cells are indicated by an arrow.

and paraffin-embedded material, or frozen sections, we could demonstrate desmin positivity in all tumors (Miettinen et al. 1982; Altmannsberger et al. 1985). In particular, less differentiated rhabdomyosarcomas constantly coexpress desmin and vimentin. Desmin is not specific for tumors of skeletal muscle origin and can also be detected in smooth muscle tumors. Myofibroblasts are desmin-negative, but such cells are positively stained by the majority of muscle-specific actin antibodies. Antibodies against titin, a high-molecular-weight constituent of sarcomeric muscles, reacted solely with rhabdomyosarcomas and did not react with leiomyosarcoma (Osborn et al. 1986a). However, the percentage of tumor cells stained by the titin antibody depends on the degree of myogenic differentiation of the rhabdomyosarcoma. A biochemical study performed by Vandekerckhove et al. (1987) demonstrates that the major component of actin in rhabdomyosarcomas belongs to the cardiac (fetal) actin type and not to the skeletal muscle type.

Recently, a study was published in which a simultaneous expression of keratin (KL1), desmin, and S-100 antigen was detected in 3 of 60 rhabdomyosarcoma cases (5%) (Coindre et al. 1988). Up to now, we have not seen such a case. It is possible that this combination of antigens is characteristic for a special subtype of neuroectodermal tumors. Additionally, keratin-positive cells are observed in normal smooth muscle, as well as in smooth muscle, tumors (Norton et al. 1987).

Nephroblastoma

Nephroblastomas are embryonal tumors of kidney and the most common kidney tumor in childhood. Nephroblastomas are characterized by three structures in light microscopy: tubuli or glomeruloid bodies, blastema, and stroma. Our immunohistological results (Altmannsberger et al. 1984) and those of others (Denk et al. 1985) demonstrate that blastema cells were labeled by antibodies to vimentin, as well as by antibodies to keratin, in the majority of cases. Tubuli in nephroblastoma could only be labeled by keratin antibodies and were negative when tested with the vimentin antibody. In the minority of cases, which lack tubuli formation by hematoxylin-eosin staining, the blastematous structures could be decorated only by the vimentin antibody and not by the keratin antibody. The clear cell sarcoma of kidney (bone-metastasizing renal tumor in childhood) could only be labeled by antibodies to vimentin. In addition, we have seen one case of malignant rhabdoid tumor of kidney and could demonstrate a positive reaction of the typical inclusion bodies with antibodies against the NF triplet, especially N52 and NE14. In contrast, rhabdoid tumors of soft tissue consistently coexpress keratin and vimentin (Vogel et al. 1984). Thus, it is likely that malignant rhabdoid tumors comprise neoplasms of different histogenesis, which have in common the globular arrangement of densely packed IFs.

In cases of nephroblastoma, we have also used antibodies specific for proximal (N4A4; Calla) and distal (BA2; Tamm-Horsfall protein) tubules (Altmannsberger et al. 1988). It becomes evident that in classic triphasic nephroblastoma, the majority of tubules have an antigenic profile according to a distal tubule, but there are some tubules expressing the phenotype of proximal tubule in all cases.

Non-Hodgkin Lymphoma

Malignant lymphomas, a primary neoplastic process of the lymphoid cells, are distinguished from myeloproliferative disorders (e.g., acute and chronic myelogenous leukemia) and histiocytosis. Non-Hodgkin's lymphoma and its categorization have been the subject of many classifications (Rappaport, Lukes and Collins, Kiel classification). In childhood, most common lymphomas are high-grade, malignant non-Hodgkin, especially lymphoblastic lymphoma. Malignant lymphomas, unlike malignant melanomas, meningiomas, and schwannomas, show variable expression of vimentin. Whereas in our experience (Altmannsberger and Osborn 1987) and that of other investigators (Gabbiani et al. 1981), the majority of tumor cells express vimentin; other workers have described the majority of malignant lymphomas as vimentin-negative (Giorno and Sciotto 1985; Azumi and Battifora 1987). In our study, we have reexamined frozen sections of 25 different low- and high-grade malignant lymphomas, using four different monoclonal antibodies against vimentin. With the monoclonal antibodies V9 and MVI, we could demonstrate a positive reaction in all the different lymphoma types independent of their T- and B-cell origin. Interestingly, when the different vimentin antibodies were compared, extensive differences in the reactivity pattern could be observed, e.g., the antibody 43βE8 did not stain any lymphoma. Although no information is available on the epitopes recognized by the different antibodies, V9 and MVI clearly recognize different epitopes. In our study, positive keratin staining was only detected in fibroblastic reticulum cells (Franke and Moll 1987).

Finally, our results suggest that the differential diagnosis of small, blue round cell tumors in childhood can be aided by the use of appropriate antibodies against intermediate filaments.

REFERENCES

Altmannsberger, M. and M. Osborn. 1987. Mesenchymal tumor markers: Intermediate filaments. *Curr. Top. Pathol.* **77**: 155.

Altmannsberger, M., K. Weber, R. Droste, and M. Osborn. 1985. Desmin is a specific marker for rhabdomyosarcomas of human and rat origin. *Am. J. Pathol.* **118**: 85.

Altmannsberger, A., M. Osborn, H.J. Schäfer, A. Schauer, and K. Weber. 1984. Distinction of nephroblastoma from other childhood tumors using antibodies to intermediate filaments. *Virchows Arch. Cell Pathol.* **51**: 265.

Altmannsberger, M., F. Wagner, H. Fitz, H.W. Birk, and M. Osborn.

1988. Differenzierung in embryonalen Tumoren. *Verh. Dtsch. Ges. Pathol.* (in press).

Azumi, N. and H. Battifora. 1987. The distribution of vimentin and keratin in epithelial and non-epithelial neoplasma. *Am. J. Clin. Pathol.* **88**: 286.

Christiansen, H. and F. Lampert. 1988. Tumor karyotype discriminates between good and bad prognostic outcome in neuroblastoma. *Br. J. Cancer* **57**: 121.

Coindre, J.-M., A. De Mascarel, M. Trojant, I. De Mascarel, and A. Pages. 1988. Immunohistochemical study of rhabdomyosarcoma. Unexpected staining with S100 protein and cytokeratin. *J. Pathol.* **155**: 127.

Denk, H., W. Weybora, M. Ratschek, R. Schar, and W.W. Franke. 1985. Distribution of vimentin, cytokeratins, and desmosomal plaque proteins in human nephroblastoma as revealed by specific antibodies: Co-existence of cell groups of different degrees of epithelial differentiation. *Differentiation* **29**: 88.

Franke, W.W. and R. Moll. 1987. Cytoskeletal components of lymphoid organs. I. Synthesis of cytokeratins 8 and 18 and desmin in subpopulations of extrafollicular reticulum cells of human lymph nodes, tonsils, and spleen. *Differentiation* **36**: 145.

Gabbiani, G., Y. Kapanci, W. Barazzone, and W.W. Franke. 1981. Immunohistochemical identification of intermediated-sized filaments in human neoplastic cells. A diagnostic aid for the surgical pathologists. *Am. J. Pathol.* **104**: 206.

Giorno, R. and C.G. Sciotto. 1985. Use of monoclonal antibodies for analyzing the distribution of the intermediate filament protein vimentin in human non-Hodgkin's lymphomas. *Am. J. Pathol.* **120**: 351.

Gould, V.E., R. Moll, I. Moll, I. Lee, K. Schwechheimer, and W.W. Franke. 1986. The intermediate filament complement of the spectrum of nerve sheath neoplasms. *Lab. Invest.* **55**: 463.

Miettinen, M., V.P. Lehto, R.A. Badley, and I. Virtanen. 1982. Expression of intermediate filaments in soft tissue sarcomas. *Int. J. Cancer* **30**: 541.

Mukai, M., C. Torikata, H. Iri, Y. Morikawa, K. Shimizu, T. Shimoda, N. Nukina, Y. Ihara, and K. Kageyama. 1986. Expression of neurofilament triplet proteins in human neural tumors. *Am. J. Pathol.* **122**: 28.

Norton, A.J., J.A. Thomas, and P.G. Isaaction. 1987. Cytokeratin-specific monoclonal antibodies are reactive with tumors of smooth muscle derivation. An immunocytochemical and biochemical study using antibodies to intermediate filament cytoskeletal protein. *Histopathology* **11**: 487.

Osborn, M., C. Hill, M. Altmannsberger, and K. Weber. 1986a. Monoclonal antibodies to titin in conjunction with antibodies to desmin separate rhabdomyosarcomas from other tumor types. *Lab. Invest.* **55**: 101.

Osborn, M., T. Dirk, M. Käser, K. Weber, and M. Altmannsberger. 1986b. Immunohistochemical localization of neurofilaments and neuron-specific enolase in 29 cases of neuroblastoma. *Am. J. Pathol.* **122**: 433.

Shaw, G., M. Osborn, and K. Weber. 1986. Reactivity of a panel neurofilament antibodies on phosphorylated and dephosphorylated neurofilament. *Eur. J. Cell Biol.* **42:** 1.

Thiele, C.J., C. McKen, T.J. Triche, R.A. Ross, P. Reynolds, and M.A. Israel. 1987. Differential protooncogene expression characterized histopathologically indistinguishable tumors of the peripheral nervous system. *J. Clin. Invest.* **80:** 804.

Vandekerckhove, J., M. Osborn, M. Altmannsberger, and K. Weber. 1987. Actin typing of rhabdomyosarcomas shows the presence of the fetal and adult forms of sarcomeric muscle actin. *Differentiation* **35:** 126.

Vogel, A.M., A.M. Gown, J. Caughlan, J.E. Haas, and J.F. Beckwith. 1984. Rhabdoid tumors of infancy contain mesenchymal specific and epithelial specific intermediate filament proteins. *Lab. Invest.* **50:** 232.

Fixatives and Proteases, Their Effect in the Demonstration of Intermediate Filaments by Immunohistochemistry

H. Battifora

Division of Pathology, City of Hope National Medical Center
Duarte, California 91010

Immunohistochemistry (IHC) has undoubtedly become the most useful ancillary test in diagnostic anatomic pathology as it permits an unprecedented level of accuracy in areas of diagnostic difficulty. These advances are, in great part, due to the availability of monoclonal antibodies (MAbs) to molecules recognized as markers of cell lineage or differentiation. Among these, the most useful and an obligatory component of virtually every diagnostic antibody panel is the intermediate filaments (Battifora 1988). However, there are problems of reproducibility between laboratories, which stem, in large measure, from inadequate specimen preparation, particularly improper tissue fixation. In this paper, some of these problems and possible solutions are discussed.

Tissue Fixation and Processing

There is no perfect fixative for IHC. Some antigenic sites are resistant to most fixatives; many are partially degraded by tissue fixation. The majority, however, are only demonstrable by IHC in frozen tissue. Thus, an ideal specimen-processing scheme should include snap freezing of samples, as well as fixation in a variety of fixatives.

Formaldehyde, the most popular of the tissue fixatives among pathologists, is unfortunately not the most suitable fixative for IHC. Although formaldehyde penetrates the tissues rapidly, paradoxically, it fixes slowly. This is because aqueous formaldehyde solutions contain less than 0.1% free formaldehyde; the remainder is in the form of methylene glycol and its polymers. Thus, dehydration of methylene glycol to release free formaldehyde takes place slowly, as free formaldehyde is scavenged by the fixation sites and additional molecules of

43

methylene glycol become available for hydration. This timed reaction can be accelerated only slightly by raising the temperature. A minimum of 24 hours are needed for complete fixation in formaldehyde, even if the tissue is very thin (Fox 1985). There is no evidence that vacuum processing or microwave radiation (Login et al. 1987) accelerates this chemical reaction in any significant way (Azumi et al., in prep.).

Formaldehyde, as well as other aldehyde fixatives, acts by producing intra- and intermolecular cross-linking of macromolecules such as proteins, glycoproteins, nucleic acids, and polysaccharides. Although the mechanisms by which formaldehyde fixation alter the antigenicity of tissues are not well understood, it is hypothesized that epitopes are "masked" by the cross-linking. Empirically, treatment of formaldehyde-fixed tissues, with proteases, could result in removal of such fixation-induced masks and make the epitope(s) available for immuno-reaction. Of course, that would only work if the epitope itself were resistant to the protease. In actual practice, such protease treatments may be helpful, indeed obligatory, for adequate IHC; often, however, they do not help or render the results unreliable (Ordonez et al. 1988). At any rate, great attention to methodological detail is demanded when proteolytic enzymes are used for IHC, and every laboratory must determine their own standards.

Nowadays, pathologists are, for many reasons, under pressure to produce rapidly. In consequence, tissues are placed in formalin for only a few hours. Fixation then proceeds in the automatic tissue processor, in the alcohol used to dehydrate the tissue. Thus, the tissues are fixed partially in formalin and partially in alcohol. Moreover, because little attention is placed to formaldehyde-fixation time, such tissues are prone to show wide variation in antigen preservation, which is the major reason for lack of reproducibility of IHC within and between laboratories.

Less commonly, tissues are left in formaldehyde for inordinate periods of time, which leads to progressive and sometimes irreversible deterioration of antigenic sites. Some antigenic sites can be recovered by increasing the protease pretreatment, as discussed below.

Alcohol fixes tissues by coagulating proteins, with penetration and fixation taking place simultaneously. With rare exceptions, most antigens that are capable of tolerating tissue fixation are better preserved in alcohol than in formalin. Fur-

44

thermore, no masking of antigenic sites is observed in alcohol-fixed tissues and no protease pretreatment is necessary. However, tissues fixed in alcohol tend to shrink appreciably more than formalin-fixed tissues, and the quality of their cytologic detail is often suboptimal. Additionally, tissue penetration is slow and requires that specimens be cut into thin slices before processing.

Supplementation with compounds to reduce shrinkage and facilitate penetration has resulted in the creation of alcohol-based fixatives, which closely mimic the morphologic quality attainable with formalin, without its deleterious effects on antigens. A good example of such fixative is Omnifix (Xenetics, Irvine, California). Tissues can be fixed completely in Omnifix in about 4 hours, and prolonged immersion in the fixative has no deleterious effect on antigens (H. Battifora, unpubl.). Carnoy's fixative and methacarn are other alcohol-based fixatives that exhibit excellent antigen preservation.

Protease Digestion in IHC
Proteolytic digestion of formaldehyde-fixed tissue may unmask a hidden antigen if the desired epitope is intact and is not itself digestible. This is often the case with monoclonal antibodies to keratins and some monoclonal antibodies to other intermediate filaments.

In our laboratory, we compared the effect of three proteases—trypsin, pepsin, and pronase—on the immunohistochemical staining of keratins with MAb AE1, an antibody to low-molecular-weight keratins widely used in paraffin sections of formalin and ethanol-fixed tissues by the ABC method (Battifora and Kopinksi 1986). Both the length of exposure to the fixative and the duration of proteolysis were varied over a wide range. Ethanol-fixed tissues showed excellent preservation of the antigenicity of keratins, and no appreciable differences in immunostaining related to the length of fixation were found. The use of proteolytic enzymes did not improve these results; on the contrary, it led to rapid tissue disintegration. Formalin-fixed epithelial tissues stained weakly or failed to stain unless they were treated with a proteolytic enzyme. The optimal length of proteolysis varied with the degree of fixation; tissues that were fixed for long periods of time in formalin required longer exposure to a proteolytic enzyme and were more resistant to digestion than were tissues that were fixed briefly. However, the optimal digestion period varied from tissue to tissue, for unclear reasons. We hypothesize that dissimilarities in the proportion of the various keratin family members expressed by different epithelia may account for variability in the number of available shared epitopes. No significant advantage of one protease over another was found in our study. However, similar unpublished studies with other antibodies performed in our laboratory did show that some enzymes were more effective than others, depending on the antibody used.

In our consulting practice, we have observed that keratin-containing neoplasms fixed in formalin occasionally failed to immunoreact with antibodies to keratins after a routine 30-minute trypsin digestion but stained readily following prolonged incubation (2–3 hr) digestion. In most of these cases, investigation revealed that the tissues had been fixed in formalin for protracted periods of time, ranging from a few days to several weeks.

Most tissues that we receive in consultation are formaldehyde-fixed, and, in the vast majority of the cases, the length of fixation is unknown. A practical approach to these cases, which we routinely employ to demonstrate any antigen proved to be enhanced by proteolytic digestion, is as follows: Sections are digested in triplicate (or more) in twofold increments of duration of digestion (e.g., 30 min, 1 hr, 2 hr) and stained together. The slide that shows the strongest immunoreactivity and least background staining is considered to be the optimal one and is used for interpretation. Overdigestion can be readily detected as it leads to loss of cytoplasmic contents. This approach allowed us to stain positively for keratins in nearly 100% of cutaneous neuroendocrine carcinomas, whereas conventional trypsinization yielded only 70% positivity (Battifora and Silva 1986).

Summary and Recommendations
It is clear that improvements in immunohistologic techniques and the availability of superior reagents have greatly refined our diagnostic accuracy as pathologists. However, attention must be devoted to improve specimen handling to guarantee optimal preservation of antigenic substances. This requires prompt fixation, avoidance of formalin, or at least coutilization of coagulating fixatives. The need for protease digestion, a double-edged sword at best, can thus be circumvented.

Finally, because many useful antigens cannot be demonstrated in fixed tissues, regardless of the fixative employed,

46

routine freezing and storing small samples of tissue is strongly recommended.

ACKNOWLEDGMENT

This work was supported by U.S. Public Health Service grant RO1-CA-37194.

REFERENCES

Battifora, H. 1988. Clinical applications of the immunohistochemistry of filamentous proteins. *Am. J. Surg. Pathol.* **12:** 24.

Battifora, H. and M. Kopinski. 1986. The influence of protease digestion and duration of fixation on the immunostaining of keratins. A comparison of formalin and ethanol fixation. *J. Histochem. Cytochem.* **34:** 1095.

Battifora, H. and E. Silva. 1986. The use of antikeratin antibodies in the immunohistochemical distinction between neuroendocrine (Merkel cell) carcinoma of the skin, lymphoma, and oat cell carcinoma. *Cancer* **58:** 1040.

Fox, C.H. 1985. Formaldehyde fixation. *J. Histochem. Cytochem.* **33:** 845.

Login, G.R., S.J. Schnitt, and A.M. Dvorak. 1987. Rapid microwave fixation of human tissues for light microscopic immunoperoxidase identification of diagnostically useful antigens. *Lab. Invest.* **57:** 585.

Ordonez, N.G., J.T. Manning, and T.E. Brooks. 1988. Effect of trypsinization on the immunostaining of formalin-fixed, paraffin-embedded tissues. *Am. J. Surg. Pathol.* **12:** 121.

A Critical Examination of the Utility of a Select Panel of Monoclonal Antibodies in the Diagnosis of Routinely Processed Undifferentiated Neoplasms

R.B. Nagle,[1] J.A. Rybski,[3] T.M. Grogan,[1] T. Hassett,[2] P. Molloy,[1] and J. Guillot[1]

Departments of Pathology[1] and Statistics,[2]
University of Arizona, Tucson, Arizona 85724

[3]Immunodiagnostics, Tucson, Arizona 85724

The application of immunohistochemistry using specific antibodies is now established in most modern pathology laboratories (Erlandson 1984; Gatter et al. 1984). Antibodies to intermediate filaments, which can delineate cell lineage, are the cornerstones of this methodologic approach (Altmannsberger et al. 1981; Moll et al. 1982; Osborn and Weber 1983; Ramaekers et al. 1983). However, many primary hospital laboratories are still experiencing difficulty in using these techniques, especially when presented with an undifferentiated neoplasm for which there is only formalin-fixed material and a limited number of antibodies available. In this study, we have attempted to evaluate critically the utility of a select panel of monoclonal antibodies (antibodies to cytokeratins [CK], vimentin [V], desmin [D], common leukocyte antigen [CLA], and S-100) when applied using standard methods to formalin-fixed, paraffin-embedded "undifferentiated neoplasms."

SUMMARY

Two anti-CK antibodies were chosen: KA4, specific for CKs 14, 15, 16, and 19 (Nagle et al. 1986), and 10.11, specific for CKs 8 and 18 (Chan et al. 1986). This range of expression was expected to react with most carcinomas on the basis of published accounts of their specific keratin content. The vimentin, desmin, CLA, and S-100 antibodies were commercially available reagents commonly used on formalin-fixed, paraffin-embedded tissues. Seventy-eight poorly differentiated neoplasms (20 large cell lymphomas, 21 melanomas, 20 carcinomas, and 17 sarcomas) were chosen in which the diagnosis was firmly established on the basis of analysis of immunotyping using fixed and snap-frozen material, morphologic study including electron microscopy, and clinical course. The panel of six antibodies (KA4, 10.11, V, D, CLA, and S-100) was used to study fixed material on these cases. When the two anti-CK results were combined (K), the analysis produced 13 phenotypic profiles (4 each for carcinoma, lymphoma, and sarcoma, and a single type for melanoma). There was minimal overlap, except for the phenotype K (0) V (+) D (0) CLA (0) S-100 (0), which was observed in five cases of lymphoma and ten cases of sarcoma. A particular problem was the finding that although all 20 lymphomas were CLA-positive on frozen tissue analysis, only 11 were detected using this CLA on the fixed specimens. Bayesian analysis (Anderson and Moore 1979) provided crude posterior probability point estimates (p), using four diagnostic groups as follows: lymphoma 0.6290303, melanoma 0.8478261, carcinoma 0.8420455, and sarcoma 0.4431818. In practice, sarcomas are usually a clinically distinct problem. If they are eliminated from the analysis, the overlap disappears and the discriminations of the panel improve to lymphoma 0.968254, melanoma 0.968254, and carcinoma 0.965833.

The panel of antibodies was next tested on a group of 904 unselected referred "problem cases." We searched our computerized data for those cases in which at least five of the six antibodies had been applied to a case previously. This produced a cohort of 133 cases, including 53 undifferentiated carcinomas, 33 sarcomas, 20 lymphomas, 7 melanomas, 8 germ cell tumors, 5 neural tumors, and 7 unclassified tumors. The missing antibodies were performed to complete the panel, and the panel's ability to predict cell lineage was determined.

Fifty-seven cases were keratin-positive, of which 29 were vimentin-negative carcinomas and 28 were vimentin-positive neoplasms, including 21 carcinomas and 7 keratin-positive non-carcinomas. This latter group included one B cell lymphoma, two paraspinal Ewing's sarcomas, two primitive neuroectodermal neoplasms, one gliosarcoma, and one unclassifiable tumor. Two of these cases were thought to represent cross-reactivity of the keratin antibodies with GFAP (gliosarcoma)

Table 1 Frequency of Phenotypes and Predictive Values

	CK	V	D	CLA	S-100	No.	p^a	p^b
Lymphoma	0	0	0	0	0	4		
	0	0	0	+	0	5		
	0	+	0	+	0	6		
	0	+	0	0	0	5		
						20	0.63	0.97
Melanoma	0	+	0	0	+	21	0.84	0.97
Carcinoma	+	0	0	0	0	17		
	+	0	0	0	+	1		
	+	+	0	0	0	1		
	0	0	0	0	+	1		
						20	0.85	0.96
Sarcoma	0	+	0	0	0	10		
	0	+	+	0	0	3		
	+	+	0	0	0	2		
	0	+	0	0	+	2		
						17	0.44	

[a]Bayesian crude posterior probability point estimates.
[b]Probability point estimates without sarcomas.

and vimentin (lymphoma). Of the 48 keratin-positive carcinomas, 3 were S-100-positive and 1 case expressed CLA.

Seventy-six neoplasms were CK-negative. Five cytokeratin-negative carcinomas were confirmed by electron microscopy identification of desmosomes; two of these showed reactivity for CK on frozen material and were clearly related to fixation-induced artifact. Of 19 lymphomas, 4 failed to react with any of the six antibodies. Of the 19 lymphomas, 11 failed to express CLA, but 4 expressed S-100. Of ten muscle sarcomas, seven expressed desmin and three did not. Of seven melanomas, all were intensely positive for vimentin and only one failed to express S-100.

DISCUSSION

This analysis reveals that a correct cell lineage could be detected in 90.2% of difficult undifferentiated cases when a small panel of six antibodies was used on formalin-fixed, paraffin-embedded samples. Of 133 cases, 2 (1.5%) revealed cross-reactivity of CK antibodies with other intermediate filaments and 5 (3.7%) failed to react but were classified using electron microscopy and an expanded panel of antibodies. Six cases (4.5%) were sufficiently undifferentiated to prevent further classification. Improvements in fixation techniques, careful selection of a limited panel of appropriately standardized antibodies, and standardization of techniques should allow this method of diagnosis to approach the 95% level of accuracy even in fixed undifferentiated cases.

REFERENCES

Anderson, B.D.O. and S.B. Moore. 1979. *Optimal filtering.* Prentice-Hall, Englewood Cliffs, New Jersey.

Altmannsberger, M., M. Osborn, A. Schauer, and K. Weber. 1981. Antibodies to different intermediate filament proteins: Cell type-specific markers on paraffin embedded human tissues. *Lab. Invest.* **45:** 427.

Chan, R., R.V. Rositto, B.F. Edward, and R.D. Cardiff. 1986. Presence of proteolytically processed keratins in the culture medium MCF-7. *Cancer Res.* **46:** 6353.

Erlandson, R.A. 1984. Diagnostic immunohistochemistry of human tumors. *Am. J. Surg. Pathol.* **8:** 615.

Gatter, K., C. Alcock, A. Heryet, K.A. Pulford, J. Heyderman, J. Taylor-Papadimitriou, H. Stein, and D.Y. Mason. 1984. The differential diagnosis of routinely processed anaplastic tumors using monoclonal antibodies. *Am. J. Clin. Pathol.* **82:** 33.

Moll, R., W.W. Franke, D.L. Schiller, B. Geiger, and R. Keppler. 1982. The catalog of human cytokeratins: Patterns of expression in normal epithelial tumors and cultured cells. *Cell* **31:** 11.

Nagle, R.B., W. Bocker, J. Davis, H.W. Heid, M. Kaufman, D.O. Lucas, and E.D. Jarasch. 1986. Characterization of breast carcinoma by two monoclonal antibodies distinguishing myoepithelial from luminal epithelial cells. *J. Histochem. Cytochem.* **34:** 869.

Osborn, M. and K. Weber. 1983. Biology of disease: Tumor diagnosis by intermediate filament typing: A novel tool for surgical pathology. *Lab. Invest.* **48:** 372.

Ramaekers, F., J. Puts, O. Moesker, A. Kant, A. Huysmans, D. Haag, P. Jap, C. Herman, and G. Vooijs. 1983. Antibodies to intermediate filament proteins in the immunohistochemical identification of human tumors: An overview. *Histochem. J.* **15:** 691.

Value of Cytoskeletal Markers in Diagnosis of Lymphomas and Other Tumors

K.C. Gatter and D.Y. Mason

Nuffield Department of Pathology, John Radcliffe Hospital
Oxford OX3 9DU, England

Antibodies to intermediate filaments are widely used in routine pathological diagnosis. This is due largely to the development of antibodies that recognize epitopes resistant to most fixation and processing protocols (Gatter et al. 1984a). This paper concentrates on their value to the practicing pathologist, with the main emphasis being on the diagnosis of lymphoma (as other tumor types will be covered comprehensively by other papers in this volume).

There are two aspects to the diagnosis of lymphoma. The first is the distinction of lymphoma from other tumor types such as carcinoma or sarcoma, and the second is the classification of lymphoma into one of the subtypes based on a variety of clinical and pathological features.

The recognition of a tumor as lymphoma forms part of the differential diagnosis of malignant tumors and is a regular task for practicing pathologists. Tumors may be of uncertain origin for a variety of reasons. Their morphological differentiation may be too primitive to allow a distinction of anything more than a malignancy, i.e., an anaplastic tumor. Another cause of diagnostic difficulty is the increasing number of small biopsies resulting from newer biopsy techniques such as endoscopy or fine needle aspiration. Here, the amount of material may be too little or too distorted to give enough architectural detail to indicate the type of tumor. For all of these reasons, malignant tumors that cannot be further specified have formed a small but constant part of the pathologist's workload for many years. Until recently, however, there was little therapy available for many of these malignancies which, particularly in the case of anaplastic tumors, were believed to behave poorly regardless of cell type of origin. With the advent of modern chemotherapeutic regimens, this situation has changed, especially with regard to lymphomas.

Table 1 Monoclonal Antibodies Used for Analysis of Routinely Processed Tissue

Antibody	Antigen[a]	Source
PD7/26,2B11	leukocyte common (CD45)	Dakopatts
E29	epithelial membrane antigen	Dakopatts
CEA	carcinoembryonic antigen	various
KL1	cytokeratin IFs	Immunotech, Dianova
CAM5.2	cytokeratin IFs	Becton-Dickinson
S1.61	S100 protein	this laboratory
NK1/C3	melanoma-associated antigen	Dakopatts
D33	desmin IFs	Dakopatts, Eurodiagnostics
V9	vimentin IFs	Dakopatts, Amersham
NF11	neurofilaments	Dakopatts, Eurodiagnostics
GF2	glial IFs	Dakopatts, Amersham

[a]IFs = intermediate filaments.

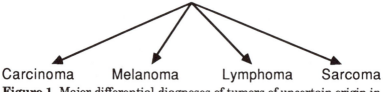

Figure 1 Major differential diagnoses of tumors of uncertain origin in adults.

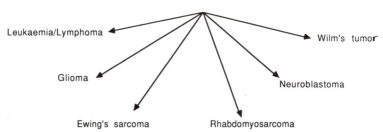

Figure 2 Principal differential diagnoses in pediatric undifferentiated tumors.

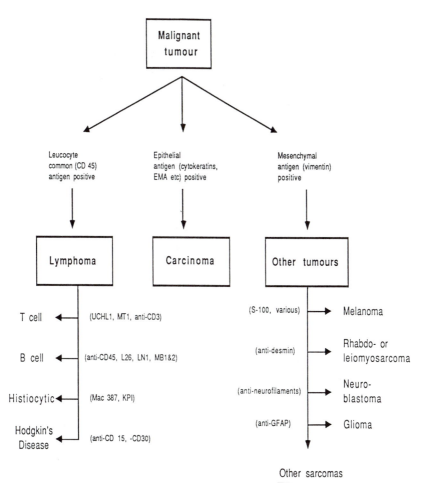

Figure 3 Differential diagnosis of malignant tumors, using a variety of monoclonal antibodies that recognize fixation-resistant antigenic epitopes. (Reprinted, with permission, from Mason and Gatter 1987.)

In the past few years, it has been shown in a number of different studies (Gatter et al. 1984b; Lauder et al. 1984; Kurtin and Pinkus 1985; Poston and Sidhu 1986; Michie et al. 1987) that a small panel of monoclonal antibodies is very useful in the distinction of tumors of unknown origin, even when only routinely processed material is available. Such a panel of antibodies, most of which are readily available from a variety of commercial sources, is indicated in Table 1.

Malignancies including anaplastic tumors are much more

Table 2 Details of Original Diagnosis and Immunostaining Results

Case No.	Initial diagnosis[a]	Monoclonal antibodies against[b]						Final conclusion
		cytokeratin	EMA	S100	LCA	vimentin	desmin	
1	anaplastic carcinoma	+	+	+	−	+	−	carcinoma
2	anaplastic carcinoma	+	+	+	−	−	−	carcinoma
3	anaplastic carcinoma	+	+	+	−	−	−	carcinoma
4	anaplastic carcinoma	−	−	+	−	−	−	melanoma
5	anaplastic carcinoma	+	+	+	−	−	−	carcinoma
6	anaplastic carcinoma	+	+	+	−	−	−	carcinoma
7	anaplastic carcinoma	−	−	−	+	+	−	lymphoma
8	anaplastic carcinoma	+	+	+	−	−	−	carcinoma
9	anaplastic carcinoma	+	+	+	−	−	−	carcinoma
10	anaplastic carcinoma	−	−	−	+	−		lymphoma
11	anaplastic carcinoma	−	*	+	−	−		melanoma
12	anaplastic carcinoma	*	*	−	−	−		probable carcinoma

	Original diagnosis						Diagnosis
13	reticulosarcoma	+			−		carcinoma
14	reticulosarcoma	−	+	−	−		melanoma
15	?carcinoma	−		+	+	−	lymphoma
16	?reticulosarcoma	−		+	+		lymphoma
17	?reticulosarcoma	−	−	+	+		lymphoma
18	?reticulosarcoma	−	−	+	+		lymphoma
19	?melanoma/NHL	−	+	−	+	+	melanoma
20	?reticulosarcoma or melanoma	−	+	−	−	−	carcinoma
21	?anaplastic carcinoma or reticulosarcoma	+	+	+	−	−	carcinoma
22	?reticulosarcoma	−		+	+		lymphoma
23	?anaplastic carcinoma or melanoma	−	−	−	−		?

[a](NHL) Non-Hodgkin's lymphoma.
[b](+) More than 10% of tumor cells positive; (−) no staining; (*) focally positive, less than 10% of tumor cells. Blank spaces indicate staining not performed due to lack of material.

common in adults than in children. The differential diagnosis is also different, as indicated in Figures 1 and 2.

Figure 3 illustrates in diagrammatic form how a panel of antibodies such as those detailed in Table 1 can be used to assist in the differential diagnoses indicated in Tables 1 and 2.

A number of pathological studies (see, e.g., Gatter et al. 1985), have now established the reliability of such panels of monoclonal antibodies as those detailed above in routine pathological practice. One of the surprising features of many of the studies of adult anaplastic malignant tumors has been the large numbers of lymphomas identified. These have accounted for 25–50% of the tumors in most of these immunocytochemical studies, which is a high proportion when compared with the fact that lymphoma accounts for less than 10% of adult malignancies as a whole. The importance of this distinction has been emphasized by clinical follow-up of many of these patients

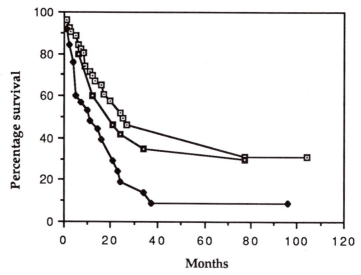

Figure 4 Survival of patients initially diagnosed as having undifferentiated tumors, which were characterized by immunocytochemical labeling. The survival of patients with lymphoma is contrasted with those having carcinoma, illustrating the better prognosis of the former (data from Robinson et al. 1988). The survival of the lymphoma patients is similar to that of patients with high-grade lymphoma from a large European series (Kiel non-Hodgkin's lymphoma [NHL]). (*Open squares*) Lymphoma; (*closed circles*) carcinoma; (*closed squares*) Kiel NHL. (Adapted from Robinson et al. 1988.)

(Robinson et al. 1988). This has not agreed with the belief previously held by many pathologists that all undifferentiated tumors have a similarly poor prognosis. In fact, as shown in the survival graph in Figure 4, the lymphomas recognized immunocytochemically behave virtually identically to the high-grade lymphomas diagnosed conventionally on morphological grounds.

With the ready availability of such panels of monoclonal antibodies, it could be argued that the traditional morphological skills of pathologists are or will be lost. To investigate this possibility, we recently recovered from our files 23 cases that had been diagnosed more than 25 years previously as anaplastic carcinoma, reticulosarcoma (the previous term for high-grade poorly differentiated lymphomas), or a differential diagnosis such as that shown in Figure 1 (S.A. Hales et al., in prep.). The results achieved from staining paraffin sections of these cases are summarized in Tables 2 and 3.

It can thus be seen that poorly differentiated tumors proved to be as difficult to diagnose to our predecessors as they do to us today. It seems clearly established, therefore, that we are justified in using a well-chosen panel of monoclonal antibodies for routine diagnosis on both pathological and clinical grounds.

Having made a diagnosis of lymphoma, the next step is to subclassify or phenotype it. Currently, this is performed with a number of antibodies against leukocyte differentiation antigens, full details of which can be found in the reports of the international conferences convened on that subject (McMichael 1987). There is as yet no identifiable role for cytoskeletal markers in the subclassification of lymphoma. Antibodies to vimentin have been applied to a number of non-Hodgkin's lymphomas in two studies. One study (Giorno and Sciotto 1985)

Table 3 Summary of Results after Immunostaining

Original diagnosis	No. of cases	C[a]	L	M	U
Anaplastic carcinoma	12	8	2	2	0
Reticulo-sarcoma	3	1	1	1	0
Differential only	8	2	4	1	1
Total	23	11	7	4	1

[a](C) Carcinoma; (L) lymphoma; (M) melanoma; (U) undiagnosed.

found only 30% positivity, with no relationship between vimentin immunoreactivity and the histological type of lymphoma. The other study (Moller et al. 1988) found vimentin staining of all lymphomas except those of germinal center origin, thus suggesting that its absence might serve as an argument for a follicular center stage of differentiation in a lymphoma. More studies are clearly needed, although it is unlikely that antibodies to vimentin will ever provide more than a small addition to the information coming from the better established leukocyte differentiation markers.

REFERENCES
Gatter, K.C., B. Falini, and D.Y. Mason. 1984a. The use of monoclonal antibodies in histopathological diagnosis. *Rec. Adv. Histopathol.* **12:** 35.
Gatter, K.C., C. Alcock, A. Heryet, and D.Y. Mason. 1985. Clinical importance of analysing malignant tumours of uncertain origin with immunohistological techniques. *Lancet* **I:** 1302.
Gatter, K.C., C. Alcock, A. Heryet, K.A. Pulford, E. Heyderman, J. Taylor-Papadimitriou, H. Stein, and D.Y. Mason. 1984b. The differential diagnosis of routinely processed anaplastic tumors using monoclonal antibodies. *Am. J. Clin. Pathol.* **82:** 33.
Giorno, R. and C.G. Sciotto. 1985. Use of monoclonal antibodies for analyzing the distribution of the intermediate filament protein vimentin in human non-Hodgkin's lymphomas. *Am. J. Pathol.* **120:** 351.
Kurtin, P.J. and G.S. Pinkus. 1985. Leukocyte common antigen—A diagnostic discriminant between hematopoietic and nonhematopoietic neoplasms in paraffin sections using monoclonal antibodies. *Hum. Pathol.* **16:** 353.
Lauder, I., D. Holland, D.Y. Mason, G. Gowland, and W.J. Cunliffe. 1984. Identification of large cell undifferentiated tumours in lymph nodes using leucocyte common and keratin antibodies. *Histopathology* **8:** 259.
Mason, D.Y. and K.C. Gatter. 1987. The role of immunocytochemistry in diagnostic pathology. *J. Clin. Pathol.* **40:** 1042.
McMichael, A., ed. 1987. *Leucocyte typing III.* Oxford University Press, Oxford, England.
Michie, S.A., D.V. Spagnolo, K.A. Dunn, R.A. Warnke, and R.V. Rouse. 1987. A panel approach to the evaluation of the sensitivity and specificity of antibodies for the diagnosis of routinely processed histologically undifferentiated human neoplasms. *Am. J. Clin. Pathol.* **88:** 457.
Moller, P., F. Momburg, W.J. Hofmann, and D.U. Matthaei-Maurer. 1988. Lack of vimentin occurring during the intrafollicular stages of B cell development characterizes follicular center cell lymphomas. *Blood* **71:** 1033.
Poston, R.N. and Y.S. Sidhu. 1986. Diagnosing tumours on routine surgical sections by immunohistochemistry: Use of cytokeratin, common leucocyte, and other markers. *J. Clin. Pathol.* **39:** 514.

Robinson, M., C. Alcock, K.C. Gatter, and D.Y. Mason. 1988. The analysis of malignant tumours of uncertain origin with immunohistological techniques: Clinical follow-up. *Clin. Radiol.* **39:** 432.

Intermediate Filament Proteins in Soft Tissue Sarcomas: New Findings Suggest a Complex Pattern of Expression

M. Miettinen

Department of Pathology, University of Helsinki, Helsinki, Finland

Since the first description of the use of a panel of antibodies to different classes of intermediate filament (IF) proteins in surgical pathology (Gabbiani et al. 1981), immunohistochemistry of IF proteins not only has represented a set of useful diagnostic tests, but has also given new insights to the cellular nature of many tumors and clarified the taxonomic relationships of many tumors, including soft tissue sarcomas (Osborn and Weber 1983; Ramaekers et al. 1983; Miettinen et al. 1984). The basis for the use of IF proteins as cell-type-specific markers in tumor diagnosis is that their expression in neoplastic cells closely parallels that of normal cells, as follows: Keratins are present in epithelial cells, vimentin in most mesenchymal cells in general, desmin in all striated and some, but not all, smooth muscle cells, neurofilament proteins in neural cells, and glial fibrillar acidic protein in glial cells (Franke et al. 1982; Osborn and Weber 1983).

Early immunohistochemical and biochemical work in the beginning of the 1980s indicated that nonmuscle sarcomas contain vimentin, muscle sarcomas contain desmin, and synovial sarcoma, as well as epithelioid sarcoma, contain keratin(s) (Altmannsberger et al. 1982; Miettinen et al. 1982; Denk et al. 1983; Chase et al. 1984). Since then, the patterns of IF expression in mesenchymal tumors have proved to be more complex than was originally thought. This has resulted, in part, from the introduction of a number of new monoclonal antibodies and use of optimal tissue material in immunostaining and, in part, from the fact that much larger tumor series have now been investigated, thus revealing the exceptions. This paper deals with the IF expression in soft tissue sarcomas, with an emphasis on keratins and is mostly based on my observations.

Synovial Sarcoma

The results pertaining to the keratin positivity of the epithelium-like cells in synovial sarcoma, originally obtained with rabbit antibodies to epidermal plantar callus keratins (Miettinen et al. 1982; Corson et al. 1984), have been fully confirmed with several monoclonal antibodies. All synovial sarcomas tested so far have been positive with the monoclonal antibodies to keratins 7, 8, 18, and 19, i.e., the whole set of simple epithelial keratins. In agreement with the true epithelial nature of the epithelium-like cells of synovial sarcoma, these cells show immunoreactivity for desmosome plaque proteins, at least for desmoplakin and desmoglein.

Leiomyosarcoma

Besides the fact that leiomyosarcomas (LMSs) have usually shown desmin and/or muscle actin immunoreactivity and that many of these tumors also contain vimentin, a number of well-documented LMSs have showed keratin immunoreactivity. In various reports, the percentage of cytokeratin positivity has varied from about 40% to nearly 100% (Brown et al. 1987; Norton et al. 1987; Miettinen 1988). The keratin positivity in LMSs has been found with different monoclonal antibodies (CAM 5.2, PKK1, AE3, 35βH11) and with different immunostaining techniques (immunoperoxidase, immunofluorescence). Furthermore, similar keratin immunoreactivity has been found in nonneoplastic smooth muscle cells in the myometrium (Huitfeldt and Brandzaeg 1985), where the presence of keratins 8 and 18 has been confirmed recently by Western blotting analysis (Gown et al. 1988).

Rhabdomyosarcoma

One of the earliest findings in the field of the use of antibodies to IF proteins in surgical pathology was that rhabdomyosarcomas (RMSs) are desmin-positive (Gabbiani et al. 1981; Altmannsberger et al. 1982; Miettinen et al. 1982). Numerous series of tumors analyzed and published thereafter have confirmed the value of desmin in the immunohistochemical diagnosis of RMS. Some well-documented RMSs have recently revealed unexpected complexity of IF patterns. A high number of alveolar RMSs, primitive variants in the spectrum of RMSs, have been found to contain keratin immunoreactive cells, up to one third of the total cell population. Such cells are, by morphology, undifferentiated and apparently do not represent morphological epithelial differentiation. In embryonal RMSs, keratin immunoreactivity is less common (Miettinen and Rapola 1989). Interestingly, the keratin positivity in these tumors appears in more differentiated rhabdomyoblast-like cells, rather than in less differentiated cells. Occasional RMSs have also been reported to be keratin immunoreactive by Coindre et al. (1988). Some embryonal RMSs have also showed scattered 68K neurofilament protein immunoreactive cells (Miettinen and Rapola 1989). In fetal tissues, cardiac muscle, as well as striated muscle of the tongue, may contain keratin immunoreactivity in some developmental stages (van Muijen et al. 1986). In view of this, the keratin expression in RMS can be thought to represent a regression to the fetal state. Both keratin and neurofilament immunoreactivity in RMS may alternatively imply, more commonly than thought previously, that these tumors represent neoplasms with multidirectional differentiation; so far, it has only been possible to detect the striated muscle component by electron microscopy, whereas no obvious ultrastructural marker has been available for the possible epithelial or neuron-like differentiation in RMS. It is of interest that Ewing's sarcoma also commonly displays keratin immunoreactivity and occasionally also neurofilament proteins (Moll et al. 1987).

Malignant Schwannoma
In these tumors, vimentin types of IF proteins have been regularly found (Gould et al. 1986). A number of malignant schwannomas have shown keratin immunoreactivity, as documented with several different monoclonal antibodies. The keratin-positive cells have not represented morphological epithelium-like differentiation but have belonged to the main spindle cell population indistinguishable from all other tumor cells. In some cases, even the majority of cells have been keratin-positive. Although the explanation for the presence of keratins in malignant schwannoma still remains open, these tumors may also represent multidirectionally differentiated neoplasms.

Poorly Defined Tumors with Multiple Differentiation Pathways
During the analysis of IF proteins in undifferentiated tumors, several remarkable cases with multiple expression of IF proteins have emerged. Some poorly differentiated childhood

small round cell tumors have showed simultaneous keratin, vimentin, neurofilament, and desmin positivity. Our findings have thus confirmed the existence of such immunohistochemically "pleomorphic" tumors, reported recently by Swanson et al. (1988). From these findings, it becomes obvious that straightforward diagnosis is not always possible on the basis of IF analysis. The taxonomic position and clinicopathological significance of these primitive multidirectional tumors should be tested in correlative immunohistochemical, ultrastructural, and clinicopathological studies.

DISCUSSION

The patterns of IF expression in soft tissue sarcomas seem to be more complex than thought previously. Keratins, in particular, have been found in a wide range of sarcomas, besides synovial and epithelioid sarcomas. Therefore, results of immunohistochemistry should still be applied with caution in diagnostic practice. For the rational clinical use of antibodies to IF proteins, a complete mapping of the immunohistochemical spectra of all tumor types will be mandatory. A panel of different antibodies, rather than a single diagnostic "marker," should be used in order to avoid misinterpretations. The use of other diagnostic procedures besides immunohistochemistry, such as electron microscopy, will still be important, either to provide an independent verification or as an adjunct procedure to solve complex problems. Finally, despite all cytoskeletal and other markers, a number of sarcomas still remain unclassified or taxonomically problematic, either because of the lack of expression of markers or because there is simultaneous expression of several lineage markers. Problems also result from the fact that the taxonomic system of soft tissue carcinomas is still incomplete.

ACKNOWLEDGMENT

This study was supported by the Finnish Cancer Research Fund and the Paulo Foundation.

REFERENCES
Altmannsberger, M., J. Treuner, A. Hölscher, M. Osborn, and K. Weber. 1982. Diagnosis of human childhood rhabdomyosarcoma by antibodies to desmin, the structural protein of muscle specific intermediate filaments. *Virchows Arch. Cell. Pathol.* **39**: 203.
Brown, D.C., J.M. Theaker, P.M. Banks, K.C. Gatter, and D.Y. Mason. 1987. Cytokeratin expression in smooth muscle and smooth muscle tumours. *Histopathology* **11**: 477.

Chase, D., F.M. Enzinger, S.W. Weiss, and J.M. Langloss. 1984. Keratin in epithelioid sarcoma: An immunohistochemical study. *Am. J. Surg. Pathol.* **8:** 435.

Coindre, J.-M., A. De Mascarel, M. Trojani, I. De Mascarel, and A. Pages. 1988. Immunohistochemical study of rhabdomyosarcoma. Unexpected staining with S100 protein and cytokeratin. *J. Pathol.* **155:** 127.

Corson, J.M., L.M. Weiss, S.P. Banks-Schlegel, and G.S. Pinkus. 1984. Keratin proteins and carcino-embryonic antigen in synovial sarcomas: An immunohistochemical study of 24 cases. *Hum. Pathol.* **15:** 615.

Denk, H., R. Krepler, U. Artlieb, G. Gabbiani, E. Rungger-Brändle, P. Leoncini, and W.W. Franke. 1983. Proteins of intermediate filaments. An immunohistochemical and biochemical approach to the classification of soft tissue tumors. *Am. J. Pathol.* **110:** 193.

Franke, W.W., E. Schmid, D.L. Schiller, S. Winter, E.D. Jarasch, R. Moll, H. Denk, B.W. Jackson, and K. Illmensee. 1982. Differentiation-related patterns of expression of proteins of intermediate-size filaments in tissues and cultered cells. *Cold Spring Harbor Symp. Quant. Biol.* **46:** 431.

Gabbiani, G., Y. Kapanci, P. Barazzone, and W.W. Franke. 1981. Immunochemical identification of intermediate-sized filaments in human neoplastic cells. A diagnostic aid for the surgical pathologist. *Am. J. Pathol.* **104:** 206.

Gould, V.E., R. Moll, I. Moll, I. Lee, K. Schwechheimer, and W.W. Franke. 1986. The intermediate filament complement of the spectrum of nerve sheath neoplasms. *Lab. Invest.* **55:** 463.

Gown, A.M., H.C. Boyd, M. Ferguson, and D. Tippens. 1988. Cytokeratin expression by myometrial smooth muscle cells in vivo and in vitro. *Lab. Invest.* **58:** 35A.

Huitfeldt, H.S. and P. Brandtzaeg. 1985. Various keratin antibodies produce immunohistochemical staining of human myocardium and myometrium. *Histochemistry* **83:** 381.

Miettinen, M. 1988. Immunoreactivity for cytokeratin and epithelial membrane antigen in leiomyosarcoma. *Arch. Pathol. Lab. Med.* **112:** 637.

Miettinen, M. and J. Rapola. 1989. Immunohistochemical spectrum of rhabdomyosarcoma and rhabdomyosarcoma-like tumors. *Am. J. Surg. Pathol.* (in press).

Miettinen, M., V.-P. Lehto, and I. Virtanen. 1984. Antibodies to intermediate filament proteins in the diagnosis and classification of human tumors. *Ultrastruct. Pathol.* **7:** 83.

Miettinen, M., V.-P. Lehto, R.A. Badley, and I. Virtanen. 1982. Expression of intermediate filaments in soft tissue sarcomas. *Int. J. Cancer* **30:** 541.

Moll, R., I. Lee, V.E. Gould, R. Berndt, A. Roessner, and W.W. Franke. 1987. Immunocytochemical analysis of Ewing's tumors. Patterns of expression of intermediate filaments and desmosomal proteins indicate cell-type heterogeneity and pluripotential differentiation. *Am. J. Pathol.* **127:** 288.

Norton, A.J., J.A. Thomas, and P.G. Isaacson. 1987. Cytokeratin-specific monoclonal antibodies are reactive with tumours of smooth muscle derivation. An immunocytochemical and biochemical study using antibodies to intermediate filament cytoskeletal proteins. *Histopathology* **11:** 487.

Osborn, M. and K. Weber. 1983. Biology of disease. Tumor diagnosis by intermediate filament typing: A novel tool for surgical pathology. *Lab. Invest.* **48:** 372.

Ramaekers, F.C.S., J.J.G. Puts, O. Moesker, A. Kant, A. Huysmans, D. Haag, P.H.K. Jap, C.J. Herman, and G.P. Vooijs. 1983. Antibodies to intermediate filament proteins in the immunohistochemical identification of human tumors: An overview. *Histochem. J.* **15:** 691.

Swanson, P.E., L.P. Dehner, and M.R. Wick. 1988. Polyphenotypic small cell tumors of childhood. *Lab. Invest.* **58:** 9P.

van Muijen, G.N.P., D.C. Ruiter, and S.O. Warnaar. 1986. Coexpression of intermediate filament polypeptides in human fetal and adult tissues. *Lab. Invest.* **57:** 359.

Melanocyte-specific Cytoplasmic and Secreted Antigens

A.M. Vogel

Department of Pathology, St. Louis University
St. Louis, Missouri 63104

Malignant melanoma occasionally presents as an undifferentiated neoplasm and can therefore be a diagnostic problem in surgical pathology. To aid in the diagnosis of melanoma, we have isolated two monoclonal antibodies, designated HMB-45 and HMB-50, that specifically recognize melanocyte-derived lesions (Gown et al. 1986; Vogel and Esclamado 1988). These antibodies recognize melanomas, junctional nevi, and fetal and neonatal melanocytes but fail to react with adult melanocytes and intradermal nevi (Table 1). Nonmelanocyte-derived normal, benign, and malignant tissues do not react with these antibodies. The specificity of these antibodies and the fact that they recognize the vast majority of melanomas make them excellent diagnostic reagents.

The specificity of these antibodies is also observed in tissue culture, where they recognize a majority of human melanoma cell lines and normal neonatal foreskin melanocytes but fail to react with a variety of carcinomas and human fibroblasts (Vogel and Esclamado 1988). Immunofluorescence experiments

Table 1 Reactivity of Melanocytic Lesions with HMB-45 and HMB-50

	Reactivity
Adult melanocytes	−
Fetal melanocytes	+
Neonatal melanocytes	+
Intradermal nevi	−
Junctional nevi	+
Dysplastic nevi	+
Atypical melanocytic hyperplasia	+
Lentigo maligna	+
Spitz tumor	+
Melanoma	+

demonstrate a granular cytoplasmic staining pattern (Gown et al. 1986; Vogel and Esclamado 1988).

Immunoprecipitation experiments show that HMB-45 detects a 10-kD peptide in extracts of melanomas and melanocytes, whereas HMB-50 reacts with a 95-kD glycoprotein in cell extracts and the growth medium (Esclamado et al. 1986; Vogel and Esclamado 1988). Pulse-chase experiments reveal that the 95-kD molecule is rapidly released into the growth medium. It therefore appears to be a secreted glycoprotein (Vogel and Esclamado 1988). Normal melanocytes and one melanoma line secrete relatively large quantities of the molecule (0.5–1 μg/10^6 cells/24 hr), which has allowed us to purify milligram quantities by antibody affinity chromatography. The melanocyte-derived molecule migrates slightly faster on SDS-polyacrylamide gels than the melanoma-derived lesion. This size difference appears to result from posttranslational modifications because short pulse experiments reveal no differences in the size of the peptide in normal and malignant cells (Vogel and Esclamado 1988).

Recent experiments have shown that the production of this glycoprotein by normal melanocytes is proliferation-dependent. Normal melanocytes are grown routinely in medium MCDB 153, supplemented with pituitary extract and TPA (Boyce and Ham 1983; Pittelkow et al. 1986). Deletion of either factor results in both cessation of growth and absence of 95-kD synthesis (data not shown). Readdition of the missing growth factor stimulates growth and production of the glycoprotein (data not shown). This proliferation sensitivity of 95-kD production may explain why the molecule is not detected in adult melanocytes or dermal nevi, as these cells may be quiescent and therefore not synthesize the molecule.

The extreme specificity of these antibodies for melanocytic lesions makes them excellent diagnostic reagents for use in surgical pathology. The specificity described here has been confirmed in studies by three other laboratories (Colombari et al. 1988; Walts et al. 1988; Wick et al. 1988), and one laboratory has isolated a monoclonal antibody with similar tissue and antigenic specificity (Venegoor et al. 1988).

When isolating these antibodies, we hoped that they would also be useful for studying melanocyte function, development, and neoplastic transformation. The 95-kD glycoprotein may be of interest in this regard because it is present in fetal and neonatal but not adult melanocytes, its production is proliferation-sensitive, and its size differs in normal and neoplastic melanocytes. We are currently examining fetal skin to determine when the antigen is first expressed in development. The function of this glycoprotein remains unknown. It is clearly unrelated to previously described melanoma-associated antigens such as P97, the transferrin-related surface glycoprotein (Brown et al. 1982), a high-molecular-weight proteoglycan (Ross et al. 1983), and a 94-kD glycoprotein secreted by melanomas and carcinomas (Natali et al. 1982; Vogel and Esclamado 1988). It does not appear to be part of the extracellular matrix nor does it affect the growth of normal melanocytes (data not shown). It is probably not involved in pigment production because it is detected in both pigmented and nonpigmented melanomas (Gown et al. 1986; Vogel and Esclamado 1988). The fact that it is secreted raises the possibility that it interacts with surrounding cells such as keratinocytes. We are currently cloning the gene encoding this glycoprotein to see whether it is related to known proteins.

REFERENCES

Boyce, S. and R. Ham. 1983. Calcium regulated differentiation of normal human epidermal keritinocytes in chemically defined clonal cultures and serum-free serial cultures. *J. Ivest. Dermatol.* (suppl.) **81:** 335.

Brown, J., R. Hewick, I. Hellstrom, K.E. Hellstrom, R. Doolittle, and W. Dreyer. 1982. Human melanoma associated P97 is structurally and functionally related to transferrin. *Nature* **296:** 171.

Colombari, R., F. Bonetti, G. Zamboni, A. Scarpa, F. Marino, A. Tomezzoli, P. Capelli, F. Menestrina, M. Chilosi, and L. Fiore-Donati. 1988. Distribution of melanoma specific antibody (HMB-45) in benign and malignant melanocytic tumours. An immunohistochemical study on paraffin sections. *Virchows Arch. A Pathol. Anat.* **413:** 17.

Esclamado, R., A. Gown, and A. Vogel. 1986. Unique proteins defined by monoclonal antibodies specific for human melanoma. Some potential clinical applications. *Am. J. Surg.* **152:** 376.

Gown, A., A. Vogel, D. Hoak, F. Gough, and M. McNutt. 1986. Monoclonal antibodies specific for melanocytic tumors distinguish subpopulations of melanocytes. *Am. J. Pathol.* **123:** 195.

Natali, P., B. Wilson, K. Imai, A. Bigotti, and S. Ferrone. 1982. Tissue distribution, molecular profile and shedding of a cytoplasmic antigen identified by the monoclonal antibody 465.12S to human cell lines. *Cancer Res.* **42:** 583.

Pittelkow, M., J. Wille, and R. Scott. 1986. Two functionally distinct classes of growth arrest states in human prokeratinocytes that regulate clonogenic potential. *J. Invest. Dermatol.* **86:** 410.

Ross, A., G. Cosso, M. Herlyn, J. Bell, Z. Steplewski, and H. Koprowski. 1983. Isolation and chemical characterization of a melanoma associated proteoglycan antigen. *Arch. Biochem. Biophys.* **225:** 370.

Venegoor, C., P. Hageman, H. Van Nouhuijs, D. Ruiter, J. Calafat, P. Ringens, and P. Rumke. 1988. A monoclonal antibody specific for cells of the melanocyte lineage. *Am. J. Pathol.* **130:** 179.

Vogel, A. and R. Esclamado. 1988. Identification of a secreted M_r 95,000 glycoprotein in human melanocytes and melanomas by a melanocyte specific monoclonal antibody. *Cancer Res.* **48:** 1286.

Walts, A., J. Said, and I.P. Shintaku. 1988. Cytodiagnosis of malignant melanoma. Immunoperoxidase staining with HMB-45 antibody as an aid to diagnosis. *Am. J. Surg. Pathol.* **90:** 77.

Wick, M., S. Stanley, and P. Swanson. 1988. Immunohistochemical diagnosis of sinonasal melanoma, carcinoma, and neuroblastoma with monoclonal antibodies HMB-45 and anti-synaptophysin. *Arch. Pathol. Lab. Med.* **112:** 616.

Actin Isoform Identification in the Diagnosis of Soft Tissue Tumors and Nonmalignant Smooth Muscle Proliferation

G. Gabbiani

University of Geneva, Department of Pathology
Centre Médical Universitaire, 1211 Geneva 4, Switzerland

Major advances in the understanding of cell differentiation and tumor characterization have been forthcoming from immunohistochemical identification of a number of antigens, particularly those associated with the cytoskeleton (Osborn and Weber 1983; Rungger-Brändle and Gabbiani 1983). The availability of antibodies specific for actin isoforms, such as α-sarcomeric (αsr) and α-smooth muscle (αsm), has made it possible to examine the expression of these proteins at the cellular level during malignant and nonmalignant conditions and to correlate the presence of these antigens with the type of malignant or nonmalignant lesion (Bulinski et al. 1983; Skalli et al. 1986). Sequencing and genetic studies have shown that at least six actin isoforms are normally expressed in warm-blooded vertebrates with a tissue-specific distribution (Skalli et al. 1987; Vandekerckhove and Weber 1978, 1979, 1981). The demonstration of the six actin isoforms requires chemical analysis of the amino-terminal tryptic peptide of actin. There are three actin isoforms having an α (acidic)-electrophoretic mobility on a two-dimensional gel: One is present in large amounts in adult skeletal muscle cells and in small amounts in cardiomyocytes; one is present in large amounts in cardiomyocytes and in minute amounts in skeletal muscle cells; and one is specific for smooth muscle cells. The β and γ spots of a two-dimensional gel correspond to two forms of actin coexpressed in all cells and are called cytoplasmic. In addition, a sixth isoform, present only in smooth muscle cells, migrates with γ-cytoplasmic actin and is referred to as γ-smooth muscle actin. With the antibodies presently available and with two-dimensional gel electrophoresis,

Table 1 Rhabdomyosarcomas: Cytoskeletal Features

Case	Indirect immunofluorescence [a]				Actin isoforms [a]		
	vimentin	desmin	αsm actin	αsr actin	α	β	γ
1	+++	++	–	++	not done		
2	++	++	–	++	+	+	+
3	+++	+++	–	+	not done		
4	++	+++	–	++	+	+	+
5	++	++	–	+	not done		
6	++	++	–	+	+	+	+
7	++	++	–	+	–	+	+
8	++	++	–	+	–	+	+
9	+++	+++	++	+	+	+	+
10	++	++	–	++	not done		
11	+++	–	–	+	–	+	+
12	++	++	–	+	–	+	+
13	+++	–	–	++	+	+	+
14	+++	++	–	++	+	+	+
15	++	–	–	++	+	+	+

[a]Intensity of fluorescence reaction: (–) Negative; (+) weak; (++) moderate; (+++) strong. Coomassie blue staining: (+) Present; (–) absent.

we have studied a series of tumors defined by means of light and electron microscopy as rhabdomyosarcomas (Skalli et al. 1988) and leiomyosarcomas, respectively (Schürch et al. 1987).

Table 2 Smooth Muscle Neoplasms: Cytoskeletal Features

Case[a]	Indirect immunofluorescence[b]				Actin isoforms[b]		
	vimentin	desmin	αsm actin	αsr actin	α	β	γ
1	++	++	–	–	–	+	+
2	++	–	–	–	–	+	+
3	++	–	–	–	–	+	+
4	+++	+	–	+	±	+	+
5	++	–	–	–	–	+	+
6	+++	–	–	–	–	+	+
7	++	–	–	++	+	+	+
8	++	+	+	–	±	+	+
9	++	++	–	–	–	+	+
10	++	++	++	–	+	+	+
11	++	+++	+++	–	+	+	+
12	+++	+++	+++	–	+	+	+
13	+++	+++	+++	–	+	+	+

[a]Cases 1–10, leiomyosarcomas; case 11, intravascular leiomyomatosis; cases 12 and 13, uterine myomas.
[b]Intensity of fluorescence reaction: (–) Negative; (+) weak; (++) moderate; (+++) strong. Coomassie blue staining: (+) Present; (–) absent; (±) present only when gel was charged with 100 μg of protein.

The results of these studies have shown that αsr actin is always present in rhabdomyosarcomas, which sometimes also express αsm actin (Table 1). In leiomyosarcomas, however, αsm actin is rarely detected, and the detection is clearly correlated with the degree of differentiation of the tumor (Table 2). Interestingly, leiomyosarcomas express αsr actin in few cases. These findings suggest that αsm actin is expressed sometime during the development of striated muscle, and αsr actin is expressed sometime during the development of smooth muscle. The first possibility has been verified during development of rat striated muscle (Woodcock-Mitchell et al. 1989). The second suggestion is under study; however, it would appear less likely, at least on the ground of philogenetic considerations.

We have also examined the distribution of αsm actin in normal soft tissues and in pathological tissues containing myofibroblasts, including normally healing granulation tissue, hypertrophic scars, fibromatoses, and stromal reaction to tumors (Skalli et al. 1986, 1989). Until now, myofibroblasts have been defined ultrastructurally as cells bearing features intermediate between those of normal in vivo fibroblasts and smooth muscle cells (Gabbiani et al. 1971; for review, see Skalli and Gabbiani 1988). Fibroblastic and/or myofibroblastic cells in these different pathological settings showed a heterogeneous cytoskeletal composition that defines four phenotypes: (1) cells expressing only vimentin (V); (2) cells expressing vimentin, αsm actin, and desmin (VAD); (3) cells expressing vimentin and αsm actin (VA); and (4) cells expressing vimentin and desmin (VD). Given this, two groups of lesions were distinguished. The first contained only V cells and consisted of normally healing granulation tissue, eschars, and normally healed scars; the second contained V cells admixed with variable proportions of VAD, VA, and VD cells and consisted of hypertrophic scars, fibromatoses, and stromal reaction to tumors (Table 3). Immunogold electron microscopy showed that αsm actin was present in a proportion of cells with ultrastructural features of myofibroblasts. These findings suggest that myofibroblasts may express varying degrees of smooth muscle differentiation during pathological situations. We do not know the mechanisms underlying the expression of smooth-muscle-specific markers in myofibroblasts, but our study may be useful for the understanding of the mechanism of normal and/or pathological wound healing and may be of prognostic value in clinical settings susceptible to contracture.

Table 3 Cytoskeletal Features of Normal Soft Tissue and Non-malignant Soft Tissue Proliferative Lesions

Tissue type	Cases	Number of cases containing			
		V cells	VA cells	VAD cells	VD cells
Normal soft tissue	10	10	0	0	0
Normally healing granulation tissue	8	8	0	0	0
Eschar	2	2	0	0	0
Normally healed scar	18	18	0	0	0
Hypertrophic scar	15	15	15	4	0
Superficial (fascial) fibromatosis[a]					
palmar	25	25	25	22	0
plantar	2	2	2	2	0
Deep (musculo-aponeurotic) fibromatosis					
extraabdominal	8	8	8	6	1
abdominal	5	5	5	4	1
Intraabdominal fibromatosis (Gardner's syndrome)	1	1	0	0	1
Stromal reaction to mammary carcinoma	10	10	10	3	0

All cases were negative for α-striated actin.
[a]Results presented are from proliferative nodules.

In conclusion, the use of antibodies specifically directed against actin isoforms may be of help for the study of development and biology of striated and smooth muscle cells, as well as fibroblasts, and for the understanding of several pathological lesions, both malignant and nonmalignant.

ACKNOWLEDGMENT

This work was supported by the Swiss National Science Foundation (grant 3.108-0.88).

REFERENCES
Bulinski, J.C., S. Kumar, K. Titani, and S.D. Hauschka. 1983. Peptide antibody specific for the amino terminus of skeletal muscle α-actin. *Proc. Natl. Acad. Sci.* **80:** 1506.
Gabbiani, G., G.B. Ryan, and G. Majno. 1971. Presence of modified fibroblasts in granulation tissue and their possible role in wound contraction. *Experientia* **27:** 549.

Osborn, M. and K. Weber. 1983. Tumor diagnosis by intermediate filament typing: A novel tool for surgical pathology. *Lab. Invest.* **48:** 372.

Rungger-Brändle, E. and G. Gabbiani. 1983. The role of cytoskeletal and cytocontractile elements in pathologic processes. *Am. J. Pathol.* **110:** 361.

Schürch, W., O. Skalli, T.A. Seemayer, and G. Gabbiani. 1987. Intermediate filament proteins and actin isoforms as markers for soft tissue tumor differentiation and origin. I. Smooth muscle tumors. *Am. J. Pathol.* **128:** 91.

Skalli, O. and G. Gabbiani. 1988. The biology of the myofibroblast: Relationship to wound contraction and fibrocontractive disease. In *The molecular and cellular biology of wound repair* (ed. R.A.F. Clark and P.M. Henson), p. 373. Plenum Press, New York.

Skalli, O., J. Vandekerckhove, and G. Gabbiani. 1987. Actin isoform pattern as marker of normal or pathological smooth muscle and fibroblastic tissues. *Differentiation* **33:** 232.

Skalli, O., G. Gabbiani, F. Babaï, T.A. Seemayer, G.P. Pizzolato, and W. Schürch. 1988. Intermediate filament proteins and actin isoforms as markers for soft tissue tumor differentiation and origin. II. Rhabdomyosarcomas. *Am. J. Pathol.* **130:** 515.

Skalli, O., P. Ropraz, A. Trzeciak, G. Benzonana, D. Gillessen, and G. Gabbiani. 1986. A monoclonal antibody against α-smooth muscle actin: A new probe for smooth muscle differentiation. *J. Cell Biol.* **103:** 2787.

Skalli, O., W. Schürch, T. Seemayer, R. Lagacé, D. Montandon, B. Pittet, and G. Gabbiani. 1989. Myofibroblasts from diverse pathological settings are heterogeneous in their content of actin isoforms and intermediate filament proteins. *Lab. Invest.* (in press).

Vandekerckhove, J. and K. Weber. 1978. At least six different actins are expressed in a higher mammal: An analysis based on the amino acid sequence of the amino-terminal tryptic peptide. *J. Mol. Biol.* **126:** 783.

―――. 1979. The complete amino acid sequence of actins from bovine aorta, bovine heart, bovine fast skeletal muscle, and rabbit slow skeletal muscle: A protein-chemical analysis of muscle actin differentiation. *Differentiation* **14:** 123.

―――. 1981. Actin typing on total cellular extracts: A highly sensitive protein-chemical procedure able to distinguish different actins. *Eur. J. Biochem.* **113:** 595.

Woodcock-Mitchell, J., J.J. Mitchell, R.B. Low, M. Kieny, P. Sengel, L. Rubbia, O. Skalli, B. Jackson, and G. Gabbiani. 1989. α-smooth muscle actin is transiently expressed in embryonic rat cardiac and skeletal muscles. *Differentiation* (in press).

Anti-actin Antibodies: Use in Diagnosis

A.M. Gown

Department of Pathology SM-30, University of Washington
Seattle, Washington 98195

Actin is one of the major components of the cytoskeleton and is ubiquitous in mammalian cells. Localized to the 7-nm microfilaments, actin is found in particularly high concentration in certain cells, e.g., muscle cells, and within certain structures of other cells, e.g., microvilli of epithelial cells. Actin is a 42-kD protein that displays microheterogeneity; i.e., there are at least six different isoforms. These isoforms can be distinguished biochemically by their differences in electrophoretic mobility and, with the use of isoform-specific monoclonal antibodies, can be demonstrated to occur in restricted sets and subsets of cells. There are four different muscle-associated actin isoforms (smooth muscle α, smooth muscle γ, cardiac α, and skeletal muscle α) and two different nonmuscle actin isoforms (nonmuscle β and nonmuscle γ). Our laboratory and several others (Gown et al. 1985; Otey et al. 1986, 1988; Skalli et al. 1986, 1988; Tsukada et al. 1987b) have generated monoclonal and polyclonal antibodies that react with overlapping subsets of these actins, according to Table 1.

Over the past 2 years, we have used one of these antibodies, HHF35, which is unique in identifying all four muscle isoforms of actin, as an aid in tissue analyses by the surgical pathologist.

Table 1 Muscle Actin in Soft Tissue Tumors

Muscle-actin-positive cells	Muscle-actin-negative cells (examples)
Rhabdomyosarcoma	Ewing's sarcoma, neuroblastoma
Leiomyoma, leiomyosarcoma	Malignant fibrous histiocytoma
Fibromatoses	Giant cell tumor
Nodular fasciitis	Angiosarcoma
Glomus tumor	Hemangiopericytoma
Gastrointestinal stromal tumor	Gastrointestinal stromal tumor

Characterization of HHF35

HHF35 is a murine IgG1, generated to a cytoskeletal extract of human cardiac muscle, which identifies a sequence in the amino-terminal portion of the actin molecule that is shared by all four muscle isoforms but not by the nonmuscle variants. Competitive ELISA studies employing synthetic peptides have demonstrated that a tripeptide sequence, V-C-D, represents at least a major portion of the epitope. Curiously, this same sequence occurs in an internal location of the β-tubulin molecule, to which the antibody will react on Western blots of SDS-PAGE preparations; in tissue sections, however, this cross-reactivity is not generally observed. Studies employing alcohol (e.g., methacarn)-fixed, as well as formalin-fixed, paraffin-embedded sections, have demonstrated that the antibody specifically identifies cardiac, skeletal, and smooth muscle cells in all tissues and in all mammalian species tested (Tsukada et al. 1987a).

Muscle Actin in Soft Tissue Processes

A principal role of HHF35 has been in the positive immunocytochemical identification of rhabdomyosarcoma from the larger subset of pediatric "small, blue, round-cell" tumors, which also include neuroblastoma, Ewing's sarcoma, lymphoma, and carcinoma in the differential diagnosis. In this regard, we have demonstrated that muscle actins are a far more sensitive marker of muscle differentiation than are traditional markers such as myoglobin and the muscle isozyme of creatinine phosphokinase (Schmidt et al. 1988). More recently, we have also compared the expression of muscle actins and the muscle-specific intermediate filament protein, desmin, in rhabdomyosarcomas and found that, in general, antibodies to muscle actins are positive in slightly more tumors than are antibodies to desmin but that the fraction of cells positive with the antibody reagents is signficantly higher, on average, with the anti-muscle actin antibody. Studies using first-trimester human fetal tissue have validated this finding by demonstrating comparable differences in muscle actin and desmin expression in developing skeletal muscle. Thus, HHF35 is a powerful reagent in the analysis of pediatric tumors, especially when placed as part of a larger antibody panel.

Owing to its cross-reactivity with smooth muscle actins, antibody HHF35 is also an important reagent in the immunocytochemical analysis of soft tissue tumors in which

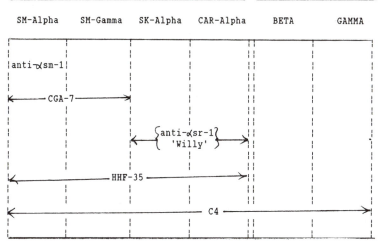

Figure 1 Actins and anti-actin antibodies. (SM) Smooth muscle; (SK) skeletal muscle; (CAR) cardiac.

leiomyosarcoma is involved in the differential diagnosis. Figure 1 summarizes our findings in soft tissue tumors.

In addition to bona fide muscle tumors (leiomyosarcomas and rhabdomyosarcomas), muscle actins have been found in tumors demonstrating "myofibroblast" differentiation. Myofibroblasts are cells of uncertain histogenesis having ultrastructural features intermediate between those of fibroblasts and smooth muscle cells and are typically found in certain healing wounds and within the stroma of certain carcinoma. Tumors demonstrating myofibroblast differentiation by ultrastructural analysis and possessing muscle actins as identified by immunocytochemical investigations employing antibody HHF35 include the family of tumors referred to as "fibromatoses," as well as curious subcutaneous skin tumors such as nodular (or proliferative) fasciitis. Identification of muscle actins in the latter can be particularly helpful in distinguishing these lesions from fibrosarcomas, which these benign, self-limited lesions can resemble histologically. Glomus cells are smooth muscle-like cells found in small organs in the skin that are thought to aid in temperature regulation; tumors of these cells (glomus tumors) have also been demonstrated to express muscle actins (although, rarely, desmin).

81

Gastrointestinal stromal tumors are a heterogeneous group of tumors, the nature of which has been controversial. Using the monoclonal antibody to muscle actins, we and others have demonstrated that a significant fraction of these tumors are positive. A variable portion of these tumors fail to react with antibody HHF35 and, instead, mark with antibodies suggestive of nerve sheath differentiation, although a third subset reacts with neither muscle nor nerve sheath markers. Soft tissue tumors that fail to demonstrate muscle actin expression include Ewing's sarcoma, malignant fibrous histiocytoma, giant cell tumor, and angiosarcoma. Curiously, we have demonstrated that the tumor categorized as "hemangiopericytoma" is devoid of muscle differentiation, as evidenced by both muscle actin and desmin expression; however, the counterpart "normal" cell, the pericyte, does express muscle actin but not desmin.

Muscle Actin Expression in Reparative Processes and Epithelial Tumors

In normal human tissues, the cell type other than muscle cells that expresses muscle actin isotypes is the myoepithelial cell, present in breast, salivary, and sweat gland, and in reparative processes, the myofibroblast, as indicated above. The presence or absence of myoepithelium can be of diagnostic significance in many proliferative and neoplastic disorders of these glands. For example, in the breast, myoepithelium is generally present along with duct epithelium in benign processes such as sclerosing adenosis and benign epitheliosis but is lost in intraductal carcinomas and infiltrating carcinomas. Distinction of tubular carcinoma from sclerosing adenosis can thus be made using antibodies to muscle actins, which are present within the myoepithelium of the latter but absent in the former; in a similar manner, benign and malignant papillary lesions can be distinguished.

In the lung, cells bearing muscle actin isotypes (outside of vascular smooth muscle cells) are rare, but increasing numbers of these cells appear in certain reparative and proliferative lung disorders. In the early phase of diffuse alveolar damage, for example, no significant increase in these cells is apparent. As the process persists, however, at some point muscle-actin-positive cells appear in increasing numbers, both in the interstitium and finally in the alveolar spaces. We hypothesize that the onset of proliferation of these cells heralds the commencement of an irreversible phase of lung injury and repair.

Cytokeratins of Simple Epithelium in Muscle Cells

The converse of muscle cytoskeletal proteins (i.e., actin) expression by certain epithelium is the curious expression of epithelial cytoskeletal proteins (i.e., cytokeratins) by smooth muscle cells. First observed in normal myometrium, it has now been observed in gut smooth muscle cells during development, prostatic muscular stromal cells, umbilical cord muscle cells, myointimal cells of atherosclerotic plaques, and in leiomyosarcomas. We have extended these studies by growing myometrial smooth muscle cells in culture and demonstrating coexpression of muscle actins and cytokeratins in the same cell, and by performing Western blots to determine that it is the simple cytokeratins (especially cytokeratin 19, but also cytokeratin 8 and possibly 18), that are anomalously coexpressed. The significance of this finding for the diagnostic pathologist is that this "anomalous" expression of cytokeratins, taken out of context, could lead to misdiagnosis of an epithelial tumor.

Significance and Future Directions

The availability of reagents such as antibody HHF35, which can be applied both prospectively and retrospectively to tissue fixed in either aldehye- or alcohol-based fixatives, affords the diagnostic pathologist a powerful tool that can be used in the characterization of human tumors by the identification of muscle differentiation in a very sensitive and specific fashion. Armed with this tool, the surgical pathologist can improve his or her diagnostic accuracy, especially in tumors in which histology alone does not offer unequivocal clues. It is also possible to test hypotheses about the "histogenesis" of various tumors and the relationship of different cell types to one another in developing neoplastic lesions. Finally, the unexpected expression of cytokeratin by muscle cells raises interesting questions about the relationship of epithelium to muscle and leads to questions, which we are currently investigating, about factors, such as estrogens or retinoids, that may be instrumental in controlling this anomalous cytokeratin expression.

REFERENCES
Gown, A.M., A.M. Vogel, D. Gordon, and P.L. Lu. 1985. Smooth muscle specific monoclonal antibodies: Specific recognition of smooth muscle actin isotypes. *J. Cell Biol.* **100:** 807.

Otey, C.A., M.H. Kalnoski, and J.C. Bulinski. 1988. Immunolocalization of muscle and nonmuscle isoforms of actin in myogenic cells and adult skeletal muscle. *Cell Motil. Cytoskeleton* **9**: 337.

Otey, C.A., M.H. Kalnoski, J.L. Lessard, and J.C. Bulinski. 1986. Immunolocalization of the gamma isoform of nonmuscle actin in cultured cells. *J. Cell Biol.* **102**: 1726.

Schmidt, R., R. Cone, J.E. Haas, and A.M. Gown. 1988. Diagnosis of rhabdomyosarcoma using HHF35, a monoclonal antibody directed against muscle actins. *Am. J. Pathol.* **131**: 19.

Skalli, O., G. Gabbiani, F. Babai, T.A. Seemayer, G. Pizzolato, and W. Schurch. 1988. Intermediate filament proteins and actin isoforms as markers for soft tissue differentiation and origin. II. Rhabdomyosarcomas. *Am. J. Pathol.* **130**: 515.

Skalli, O., P. Ropriz, A. Trzeciak, G. Benzonana, D. Gillessen, and G. Gabbiani. 1986. A monoclonal antibody against α-smooth muscle actin: A new probe for smooth muscle differentiation. *J. Cell Biol.* **103**: 2787.

Tsukada, T., M.A. McNutt, R. Ross, and A.M. Gown. 1987a. HHF35, a muscle-actin-specific monoclonal antibody. II. Reactivity in normal, reactive, and neoplastic human tissues. *Am. J. Pathol.* **127**: 389.

Tsukada, T., D. Tippens, D. Gordon, R. Ross, and A.M. Gown. 1987b. HHF35, a muscle-actin-specific monoclonal antibody. I. Immunocytochemical and biochemical characterization. *Am. J. Pathol.* **126**: 51.

Tropomyosin Gene Structure, Expression, and Regulation

D.M. Helfman, J. Lees-Miller, L. Goodwin, S. Erster, and L.A. Finn

Cold Spring Harbor Laboratory
Cold Spring Harbor, New York 11724

Tropomyosin Isoform Diversity

Tropomyosins comprise a family of related actin-binding proteins present in muscle (skeletal, cardiac, and smooth) and nonmuscle cells. Although they are present in all cells, different isoforms of the protein are characteristic of specific cell types. On the basis of migration on one- and two-dimensional polyacrylamide gel, multiple forms (or isoforms) have been detected in different tissues and cell types. Skeletal muscle contains two primary isoforms, termed α and β, the proportions of which vary with fiber type (e.g., slow- vs. fast-twitch fibers). Cardiac muscle of small animals such as rodents and chickens contains a single isoform, termed α, whereas human cardiac muscle contains at least two isoforms of tropomyosin. Smooth muscle contains at least two isoforms of tropomyosin, termed α and β. Nonmuscle tissue also contains multiple isoforms of tropomyosin. In addition, cultures of nonmuscle cells, such as fibroblasts (chicken, mouse, rat, and human), contain five to seven identifiable isoforms of tropomyosin (Matsumura et al. 1983; Hendricks and Weintraub 1984; Lin et al. 1984,1985). The functional significance of tropomyosin isoform diversity at the cellular level is not fully understood. In skeletal muscle and cardiac muscle, tropomyosin functions in association with the troponin complex (troponins I, T, and C) to regulate the calcium-sensitive interaction of actin and myosin. In contrast, the biological functions of smooth muscle and nonmuscle tropomyosins are not clearly understood. These cells are devoid of a troponin complex, and the phosphorylation of the light chains of myosin by the enzyme myosin light chain kinase appears to be the major calcium-sensitive regulatory mechanism controlling the interaction of actin and myosin. These differences in the regulation of the contractile apparatus of various cell types appear to require structurally, as well as functionally, distinct

85

forms of tropomyosin. Amino acid and nucleic acid analyses of tropomyosins from skeletal muscle, cardiac muscle, smooth muscle, and nonmuscle cells show that these proteins are highly conserved (for references, see Yamawaki-Kataoka and Helfman 1987). Nevertheless, structural differences do exist among the various protein isoforms. These divergent regions appear to correspond to functional domains of the proteins, including troponin-binding regions, actin-binding sites, and sequences involved in head-to-tail polymerization.

Nonmuscle and Muscle Isoforms Are Generated from the Same Genes by Alternative RNA Processing

Our work and that of others has revealed that the same genes encoding rat fibroblast tropomyosins also encode tropomyosin isoforms expressed in muscle (skeletal, cardiac, and smooth) and various nonmuscle tissues via tissue-specific alternative RNA-processing mechanisms. These studies have demonstrated that three genes encode at least six different polypeptides expressed in rat fibroblasts. One gene encodes rat fibroblast TM-1 and skeletal muscle β-tropomyosin via alternative RNA processing (Helfman et al. 1986). Similarly, we have determined that a second gene encodes rat fibroblast TM-2, TM-3, TM-5a, and TM-5b, as well as skeletal muscle α-tropomyosin (L. Goodwin et al., in prep.). This gene not only utilizes alternative exons for the generation of tropomyosin isoform diversity, but also contains two alternative promoters to generate at least nine different tropomyosin isoforms (J. Lees-Miller et al., in prep.). We have characterized a third gene in the rat that encodes rat fibroblast TM-4. At present, we do not know whether this gene expresses more than one tropomyosin isoform via tissue-specific RNA processing. Thus far, we have established that in the rat, at least 12 different tropomyosin isoforms are expressed from three different genes.

Alternative RNA splicing for the generation of tropomyosin isoform diversity appears to be a fundamental mechanism conserved throughout evolution because it has been characterized in various species, including *Drosophila*, chicken, quail, rat, and human (for references, see Helfman et al. 1988). In addition, the generation of protein isoforms by alternative RNA processing has been reported for other contractile protein genes, including myosin light chain, troponin T, and myosin heavy chain (for references, see Breitbart et al. 1987). Alternative RNA processing for the generation of protein isoform diversity is not restricted to contractile proteins and has been reported for a number of other proteins (for review, see Leff et al. 1986; Breitbart et al. 1987). In cases where multiple genes are differentially spliced in a tissue-specific or cell-type-specific manner, such as in muscle differentiation, it will be of considerable interest to determine whether alternative splicing of different genes is accomplished by common or gene-specific factors. For example, because the two genes that encode skeletal muscle α- and β-tropomyosins are alternatively spliced in other cell types, it will be of interest to determine whether the tissue-specific processing patterns of both genes are regulated by separate factors. In addition, smooth muscle expresses the same isoform as rat fibroblast TM-1 (Helfman et al. 1986). Understanding the mechanism by which different mRNAs arise from the various tropomyosin genes has important implications for muscle gene regulation and determination of cell type (e.g., smooth vs. skeletal). The mechanisms by which expression of different proteins are turned off and on during myogenesis are not known. When myoblasts differentiate and fuse to form myotubes, there is repression of TM-1 and TM-2 synthesis with induction of skeletal muscle β- and α-tropomyosins. Understanding the various levels of control involved in tropomyosin gene expression will provide valuable clues to understanding general mechanisms of gene regulation in a wide variety of biological systems.

Expression of Tropomyosin in Transformed Cells

Transformation of cells in tissue culture results in a variety of cellular changes, including alterations in cell growth, adhesiveness, motility, morphology, and organization of the cytoskeleton. Morphological changes are perhaps the most readily apparent feature of transformed cells. These changes in cell shape are clearly associated with the cytoskeleton. A number of groups have analyzed the expression of the protein components of microfilaments before and after transformation. Comparative two-dimensional protein gel analysis of normal and transformed cells has revealed that of the numerous cytoskeletal proteins, tropomyosin expression is selectively altered in transformed cells (Leonardi et al. 1982; Matsumura et al. 1983; Hendricks and Weintraub 1984; Lin et al. 1984,1985; Cooper et al. 1985; Leavitt et al. 1986; Takenaga et al. 1988). In general, these studies reveal that in transformed cells, one or more of the major tropomyosin isoforms of higher molecular weight are decreased or absent, whereas the levels of one or more of the low-molecular-weight tropomyosin isoforms are increased. These alterations in tropomyosin expression appear to correlate with the alterations in microfilament bundles and morphological alterations in transformed cells, although it remains to be determined whether these changes in tropomyosin expression are causally or temporally related to the changes in cell shape and cytoarchitecture. The alterations in tropomyosin synthesis have been reported to occur in cells transformed by a variety of agents, including chemical carcinogens, UV radiation, and DNA and RNA tumor viruses. In addition, the changes in tropomyosin expression following transformation occur in cells of all species examined, including chicken, rodents (mouse and rat), and man. Collectively, these results indicate that alterations in tropomyosin expression are a common feature of the transformed phenotype and that tropomyosin genes may represent a target for oncogene action.

DISCUSSION

As described above, tropomyosin isoform diversity results from the expression of multiple genes, some of which express more than one isoform by the use of alternative exons and multiple promoters. The expression of the different gene products is cell-type-specific and tissue-specific. These differences between tropomyosin isoforms may offer an opportunity for obtaining isoform-specific antibodies. The development of isoform-specific antibodies will be useful for following the expression of tropomyosin isoforms during development and in pathological processes involving these proteins. In addition, it may be possible to use these antibodies to help in the identification of certain tumor cells. At present, many questions remain concerning the functional significance and mechanisms responsible for the tissue- and cell-type-specific expression of the various isoforms. Studies of tropomyosin expression in transformed cells will provide important information concerning the role of tropomyosin expression in the transformed phenotype and provide new insights into the role of the cytoskeleton in growth control.

ACKNOWLEDGMENTS

This work was supported in part by U.S. Public Health Service grants CA-40599 and CA-46370 from the National Institutes of Health and a grant from the Muscular Dystrophy Association to D.M.H. J.L.-M. is the recipient of a postdoctoral fellowship from the Muscular Dystrophy Association.

REFERENCES

Breitbart, R.E., A. Andreadis, and B. Nadal-Ginard. 1987. Alternative splicing: A ubiquitous mechanism for the generation of multiple protein isoforms from single genes. *Annu. Rev. Biochem.* **56:** 467.

Cooper, H.L., N. Feuerstein, M. Noda, and R.H. Bassin. 1985. Suppression of tropomyosin synthesis, a common biochemical feature of oncogenesis by structurally diverse retrovirus oncogenes. *Mol. Cell. Biol.* **5:** 972.

Helfman, D.M., W.M. Ricci, and L.A. Finn. 1988. Alternative splicing of tropomyosin pre-mRNAs in vitro and in vivo. *Genes Dev.* **2:** 1627.

Helfman, D.M., S. Cheley, E. Kuismanen, L.A. Finn, and Y. Yamawaki-Kataoka. 1986. Nonmuscle and muscle tropomyosin isoforms are expressed from a single gene by alternative splicing and polyadenylation. *Mol. Cell. Biol.* **6:** 3582.

Hendricks, M. and H. Weintraub. 1984. Multiple tropomyosin polypeptides in chicken embryo fibroblasts: Differential repression of transcription by Rous sarcoma virus transformation. *Mol. Cell. Biol.* **4:** 1823.

Leavitt, J., G. Latter, L. Lutomski, D. Goldstein, and S. Burbeck. 1986. Tropomyosin isoform switching in tumorigenic human fibroblasts. *Mol. Cell. Biol.* **6:** 2721.

Leff, S.E., M.G. Rosenfeld, and R.M. Evans. 1986. Complex transcriptional units: Diversity in gene expression by alternative processing. *Annu. Rev. Biochem.* **55:** 1091.

Leonardi, C.L., R.H. Warren, and R.W. Rubin. 1982. Lack of tropomyosin correlates with the absence of stress fibers in transformed kidney cells. *Biochim. Biophys. Acta* **720:** 154.

Lin, J.J.-C., S. Yamashiro-Matsumura, and F. Matsumura. 1984. Microfilaments in normal and transformed cells: Changes in the multiple forms of tropomyosin. *Cancer Cells* **1:** 57.

Lin, J.J.-C., D.M. Helfman, S.H. Hughes, and C.-S. Chou. 1985. Tropomyosin isoforms in chicken embryo fibroblasts: Purification, characterization and changes in Rous sarcoma virus-transformed cells. *J. Cell Biol.* **100:** 692.

Matsumura, F., J.J.-C. Lin, S. Yamashiro-Matsumura, G.P. Thomas, and W.C. Topp. 1983. Differential expression of tropomyosin forms in the microfilaments isolated from normal and transformed rat cultured cells. *J. Biol. Chem.* **258:** 13954.

Takenaga, K., Y. Nakamura, and S. Sakiyama. 1988. Differential expression of a tropomyosin isoform in low- and high-metastatic Lewis lung carcinoma cells. *Mol. Cell. Biol.* **8:** 3934.

Yamawaki-Kataoka, Y. and D.M. Helfman. 1987. Isolation and characterization of cDNA clones encoding a low molecular weight nonmuscle tropomyosin isoform. *J. Biol. Chem.* **262:** 10791.

Regulation of Smooth-muscle-specific Myosin Light Chain-2 Isoform by Oncogenes

C.C. Kumar,[1] S.Mohan,[1] C. Chang,[2] and J.I. Garrels[2]

[1]Department of Tumor Biology, Schering Research
Bloomfield, New Jersey 07003

[2]Cold Spring Harbor Laboratory
Cold Spring Harbor, New York 11724

Myosin is a hexameric protein consisting of two heavy chains (MHCs) and two pairs of light chains (MLCs). Two of these light chains are classified as phosphorylatable regulatory light chains (MLC-2), and the other two are nonphosphorylatable alkali light chains (MLC-1 or MLC-3) (Kumar and Siddiqui 1988). MLC-2 is a 20,000-molecular-weight protein that plays an important role in the regulation of both smooth muscle and nonmuscle contraction (Adelstein 1983). Phosphorylation of MLC-2 by the enzyme MLC-kinase, in the presence of calcium and calmodulin, increases actin-activated myosin ATPase activity, which is critical for contraction process in smooth and nonmuscle cells. In nonmuscle cells, phosphorylation of MLC-2 also induces the assembly of myosin into ordered bipolar filaments. Together with actin, myosin forms the main component of the actin cable or microfilament network in nonmuscle cells.

Neoplastic transformation of mammalian cells leads to a dramatic change in their shape and cytoarchitecture, including the organization of the actin/myosin-containing microfilament system (Pollack et al. 1975). Cells lose the ability to assemble cytoskeletal actin cables after neoplastic transformation induced by oncogenic viruses or chemical carcinogens. The molecular mechanisms responsible for the reorganization of cytoskeletal network in transformed cells have not been understood.

Human Smooth-muscle-specific MLC-2 Isoform
We have recently isolated and characterized a cDNA clone corresponding to the human smooth muscle MLC-2 isoform from a

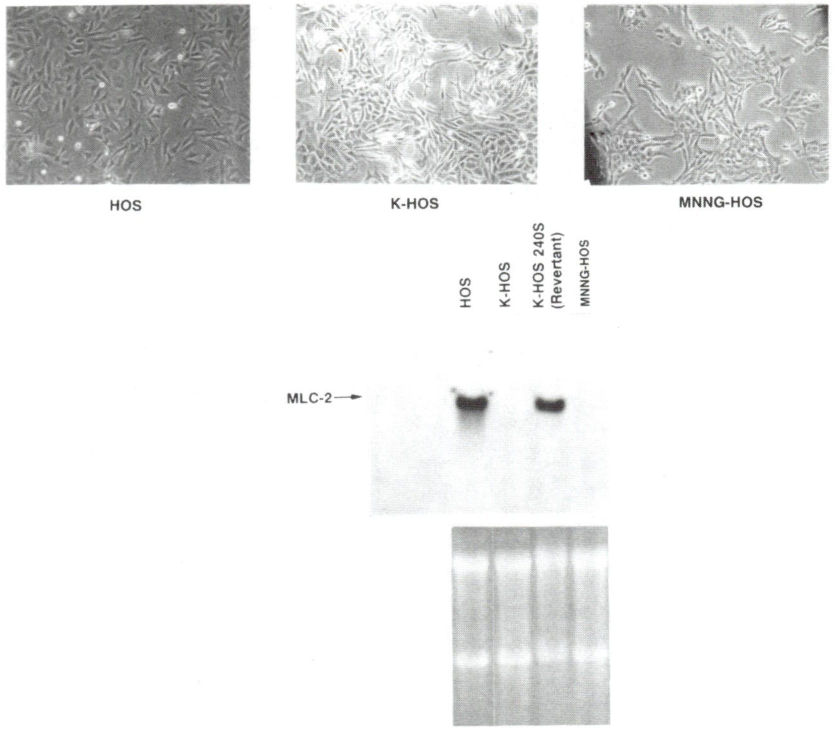

Figure 1 *(See facing page for legend.)*

cDNA library derived from umbilical artery RNA (Kumar et al. 1989). Blot hydridizations and nuclease S1 analysis indicate that this MLC-2 isoform is specifically expressed only in smooth muscle but not in other muscle tissues and also in some, but not all, nonmuscle cells. Previously reported MLC-2 cDNA (Taubmann et al. 1987), from rat aortic smooth muscle cells in culture, was found to be ubiquitously expressed in all muscle and nonmuscle cells, leading to the suggestion that both smooth muscle and nonmuscle MLC-2 isoforms are identical and are probably encoded by the same gene. In contrast, the MLC-2 cDNA that we have characterized from an intact smooth muscle tissue is expressed restrictively in smooth muscle tissues. Two-dimensional gel analysis of MLC-2 protein in human fibroblast cell lines, following immunoprecipitation using antiserum raised against purified bovine aortic MLC-2, indicates the presence of at least three MLC-2 isoforms. It appears that some nonmuscle cell lines, such as fibroblast cell lines, express one smooth-muscle-specific isoform and perhaps two or more nonmuscle MLC-2 isoforms. Other cell lines, such as hematopoietic cell lines, express only the nonmuscle isoforms (C.C. Kumar et al., in prep.).

Smooth-muscle-specific MLC-2 Isoform Is Repressed in Transformed Cells

To examine the expression of the smooth-muscle-specific MLC-2 isoform in transformed cell lines, we have used the human osteosarcoma-derived fibroblast cells known as the HOS cell line. HOS cells exhibit flat morphology and can undergo morphological transformation following treatment with chemical carcinogens, like MNNG (N-methyl-N-nitro-N-nitrosoguanidine) or oncogenic (murine) Kirsten (Ki) sarcoma virus (Rhim et al. 1975a,b). The parental HOS cells are not tumorigenic, whereas the transformed HOS sublines, such as MNNG-HOS and K-HOS, are tumorigenic (Cooper et al. 1984). Two revertant derivatives of K-HOS, known as K-HOS 240S and K-HOS 321H, were isolated that lack the v-Ki-*ras* oncogene sequences

Figure 1 Northern blot analysis of the RNAs isolated from HOS cell lines, using smooth-muscle-specific MLC-2 cDNA probe. Total RNAs (10 µg) isolated from HOS cells were electrophoresed on formaldehyde-agarose gels, transferred to Gene-screen membrane, and hybridized to radiolabeled MLC-2 cDNA insert. (*Top*) Phase-contrast micrographs of HOS, K-HOS, and MNNG-HOS cells.

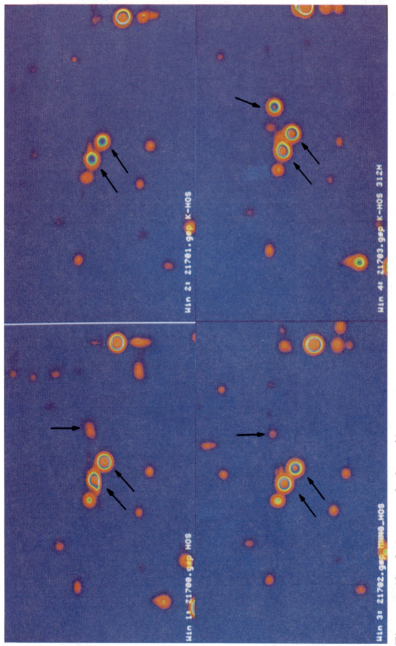

Figure 2 (*See facing page for legend.*)

and are similar to the parental HOS cell line (Cho et al. 1976; Yang et al. 1979). Northern blot analysis of HOS cell lines, using the human smooth muscle MLC-2 cDNA as a probe, indicates that MLC-2 mRNA is completely repressed in transformed K-HOS and MNNG-HOS cells (Fig. 1). The revertant of the K-HOS cell line, K-HOS 321H, expresses normal levels of MLC-2 mRNA as the HOS cells do. Similarly, a number of transformed human breast cell lines, such as SKB-3 (containing amplified *neu* oncogene sequences) and MCF-7, do not express smooth-muscle-specific MLC-2 mRNA (data not shown). Treatment of quiescent HOS cells with tumor-promoting phorbol ester, such as TPA (12-*O*-tetradecanoylphorbol-13-acetate), also results in the complete suppression of MLC-2 mRNA level in about 12–24 hours (data not shown).

Two-dimensional gel analysis of MLC-2 species from the HOS cell line indicated the presence of three MLC-2 isoforms. To identify the smooth-muscle-specific MLC-2 isoform on two-dimensional gels, we subcloned the MLC-2 cDNA insert into pGEM vectors containing the SP6 RNA polymerase promoter, and the in vitro derived transcript was translated in rabbit reticulocyte lysate systems in the presence of [^{35}S]methionine. The in vitro synthesized MLC-2 protein species was coelectrophoresed, along with the total HOS cell proteins, to identify the smooth-muscle-specific isoform in the two-dimensional gel system. Quantitative two-dimensional gel analysis of the HOS cell lines (shown in Fig. 2) indicates that the smooth-muscle-specific MLC-2 isoform is suppressed maximally in transformed K-HOS and MNNG-HOS cells.

DISCUSSION

Analysis of HOS cell lines, using smooth-muscle-specific MLC-2 cDNA and the quantitative two-dimensional gel analysis system, indicates that the smooth muscle MLC-2 isoform is repressed in transformed cells. This repression appears to be at the level of transcription. Revertants of K-HOS cells lacking

Figure 2 Quantitative two-dimensional gel analysis of the transformed (K-HOS and MNNG-HOS) and untransformed (HOS and K-HOS 312H) cell lines. Cells were labeled with [^{35}S]methionine, and total protein extracts were analyzed by two-dimensional gel electrophoresis. Fluorographs of gels were analyzed using the QUEST computer facility.

v-Ki-*ras* oncogene sequences express normal levels of MLC-2 mRNA, suggesting that activated *ras* oncogene can specifically affect the transcription of the MLC-2 gene.

A number of similarities between the actin and MLC-2 gene expression in nonmuscle cells can be noted. Nonmuscle cells express one smooth-muscle-specific (α-actin) isoform and two cytosolic or nonmuscle isoforms (β and γ). The synthesis of smooth-muscle-specific α-actin is growth-regulated and like the smooth-muscle-specific MLC-2 is also highly repressed in transformed cells (Franza and Garrels 1984). To understand the molecular mechanisms that account for the repression of MLC-2 gene expression in transformed cells, we are currently characterizing the genomic clones of MLC-2. It would be interesting to characterize the *cis*- and *trans*-acting factors that confer responsiveness to *ras* and TPA.

ACKNOWLEDGMENTS

We thank Dr. Paul Kirschmeier for introducing us to the HOS cell system and for the many valuable suggestions he has made. We wish to thank Dr. Claude Nash and Dr. Earl Ruley for support and encouragement. This work was carried out, in part, at the QUEST facility for the computer-analyzed two-dimensional electrophoresis, which is supported by grant RR02188 from the division of Research Resources of the National Institutes of Health. We thank Heidi Sacco for performing the two-dimensional gel electrophoresis.

REFERENCES

Adelstein, R.S. 1983. Regulation of contractile proteins by phosphorylation. *J. Clin. Invest.* **72:** 1863.

Cho, H.Y., E.C. Cutchins, J.S. Rhim, and R.J. Huebner. 1976. Revertants of human cells transformed by murine sarcoma virus. *Science* **194:** 951.

Cooper, C.S., D.G. Blair, M.K. Oskarrson, M.A. Tainsky, L.A. Eader, and G.F. Vande Woude. 1984. Characterization of human transforming genes from chemically transformed, teratocarcinoma, and pancreatic carcinoma cell lines. *Cancer Res.* **44:** 1.

Franza, B.R. and J.I. Garrels. 1984. Transformation-sensitive proteins of REF-52 detected by computer-analyzed two-dimensional gel electrophoresis. *Cancer Cells* **1:** 137.

Kumar, C.C. and M.A.Q. Siddiqui. 1988. Molecular genetics and control of contractile proteins. In *Molecular biology and immunology of cardiovascular diseases* (ed. C.J. Spry), p. 3., MTP Press, Lancaster, England.

Kumar, C.C., S. Mohan, P. Zavodny, S. Narula, and P. Liebowitz.

1989. Characterization and differential expression of human vascular smooth muscle myosin light chain-2 isoform in non-muscle cells. *Biochemistry* (in press).

Pollack, R., M. Osborn, and K. Weber. 1975. Patterns of organization of actin and myosin in normal and transformed non-muscle cells. *Proc. Natl. Acad. Sci.* **72:** 994.

Rhim, J.S., H.Y. Cho, and R.J. Huebner. 1975a. Non-producer human cells induced by murine sarcoma virus. *Int. J. Cancer* **15:** 23.

Rhim, J.S., C.M. Kim, P. Armstein, R.J. Huebner, E.K. Weisburger, and W. Nelson-Rees. 1975b. Transformation of human osteosarcoma cells by a chemical carcinogen. *J. Natl. Cancer Inst.* **55:** 1291.

Taubmann, M.B., J.W. Grant, and B. Nadal-Ginard. 1987. Cloning and characterization of mammalian myosin regulatory light chain (RLC) cDNA. The RLC gene is expressed in smooth, sarcomeric and non-muscle tissues. *J. Cell. Biol.* **104:** 1505.

Yang, Y.H., J.S. Rhim, S. Rasheed, V. Klement, and P. Roy-Burman. 1979. Reversion of Kirsten sarcoma virus transformed human cells: Elimination of the sarcoma virus nucleotide sequences. *J. Gen. Virol.* **43:** 447.

Differential Expression of Keratins as Seen by Monoclonal Antibodies: A Possible Function for Keratin 19

P. Stasiak,[1] X. Lu,[1] P. Morgan,[2] I. Leigh,[3] and B. Lane[1]

[1]Imperial Cancer Research Fund Clare Hall Laboratories
South Mimms, Potter's Bar
Hertfordshire EN6 3LD, United Kingdom

[2]Department of Oral Medicine and Pathology, Guy's Hospital
London SE1 9RT, United Kingdom

[3]Department of Dermatology, The London Hospital, Whitechapel
London E1 6BB, United Kingdom

The heterogeneity of the intermediate-filament-like protein gene family makes it an appropriate system for immunological analysis. Three quarters of the intermediate filament protein species identified in human tissues are (cyto)keratins, the type-I and type-II intermediate filament groups. These are characteristically expressed in epithelial cells, and different type-I/type-II pairs are expressed in different kinds of epithelia. Our approach to the question of how these keratins function differentially is based on the use of monoclonal antibodies as markers for monitoring protein expression in situ or in tissue culture situations. Of the 40 or so human keratin polypeptides, we have recently concentrated on the smallest one, keratin 19, because its apparently defective structure, together with its wide tissue distribution, should yield information about the relevance of molecular domains.

OBSERVATIONS
Immunohistochemistry
Using an extensive collection of monoclonal antibodies to keratins for immunoperoxidase staining of unfixed frozen sections of a wide variety of normal human tissues, we can now directly map the keratin phenotype of most tissues in situ, such

as we have recently done in oral epithelia (Morgan et al. 1987). These studies can reveal aspects of keratin expression that had escaped detection in earlier biochemical studies, usually because a small number of cells are involved and their keratins would be greatly diluted in a total tissue extract. An example of this is the presence of keratin 19 in the cells of the hair follicle.

The type-I keratin 19 is the smallest human keratin at 40,000 daltons on an SDS gel (Wu and Rheinwald 1981) and is usually regarded as characteristically expressed in simple epithelia (e.g., see Sun et al. 1984), although it is also expressed in significant quantities in many stratified squamous epithelia (Bartek et al. 1986). Keratin 19 is expressed in basal keratinocytes in the outer root sheath of the hair follicles, particularly around the attachment point of the *arrector pili* smooth muscle (Stasiak et al. 1988). Where the hair follicles are small, as in eyelid or forearm body skin, only a few positive cells are seen in this region with any of several antibodies to keratin 19 (listed below), but the staining is quite extensive in the large follicles of the scalp and may extend down to the hair bulb. These patterns of keratin 19 distribution are established from the earliest stages of hair follicle formation in human embryonic skin. From other studies, we have obtained evidence that this population of cells in the follicle is expanded during epidermal regeneration (i.e., more keratin-19-positive cells and altered shape of the follicle) (E.B. Lane et al., in prep.). The existence of these cells is of particular interest, as it is known that the hair follicle contains a potent progenitor population. Although keratin 19 expression is probably not an indicator of a stem cell itself, these data and other data on keratin 19 expression in the mammary gland (Bartek et al. 1985) could suggest that keratin 19 may be present in the vicinity of stem-cell populations.

We have subsequently reassessed the distribution of keratin 19 in human epithelia, using several monoclonal antibodies against keratin 19: LP2K (Stasiak et al. 1988), BA16 and BA17 (Bartek et al. 1985), A53-B/A2 (Karsten et al. 1985), and KM 4.62 (Gigi-Leitner and Geiger 1986). Quantitative differences only were observed in the staining potential of these antibodies such that KM 4.62>LP2K>BA16>BA17, in decreasing order of strength. Keratin 19 expression in stratified squamous epithelia is normally limited to the basal cell layer (Bartek et al. 1986; Gigi-Leitner et al. 1986), i.e., the compartment containing the stem cells and most of the proliferative activity of the tissue. In unfixed frozen tissue sections of several normal human tissues, we observed that keratin 19 staining appears in regions where keratin expression patterns are labile or variable, particularly in the regions near transitions between stratified epithelia and simple epithelia and in simple and stratified epithelia where more than one epithelial type or keratin phenotype appears in close proximity. This wide tissue distribution across both simple and stratified epithelial cells distinguishes keratin 19 from other human keratins and emphasizes its uniqueness among the keratins.

Sequence Analysis

We used the monoclonal antibody LP2K to clone keratin 19 cDNA from an expression library of human placenta (simple epithelium) and sequenced a 1394-bp clone containing a full-length coding region (Stasiak and Lane 1987) for a 400-amino-acid protein of 44.1 kD predicted molecular mass, with a potential glycosylation site at amino acid 393. The sequence predicted from the DNA is very like the homologous bovine sequence (Bader et al. 1986) and probably identical to another sequence for human keratin 19 from keratinocytes (see Eckert 1988); thus, there is probably only one functional gene for human keratin 19. Like the bovine amino acid sequence, keratin 19 has a truncated carboxy-terminal domain of only 13 amino acids beyond the conserved helix termination peptide TYR[X]LLEG[Q/E], and structural predictions suggest that this stretch could continue the α-helical conformation of the rod domain.

The human and bovine keratin 19 sequences are very similar, both at the DNA level and predicted amino acid level. The amino acid sequences are 86% identical over the amino-terminal head domain and 91% identical over the consensus rod domain; beyond this, however, fewer than half of the amino acid residues are shared. (Amino acid identity over any similar-length stretch elsewhere in the sequence only drops to 69%.) This suggests that the short carboxy-terminal extension is not under the same evolutionary selection pressure in the two species: Either the domains have different functions in the two species or (more likely) there is no selection pressure conserving this sequence because this piece of the molecule is nonfunctional. The alternative of no functional tail domain in keratin 19 is further supported by the recent finding of two keratin 19 sequences in *Xenopus*, which are even shorter and more divergent (Franz 1987).

No other human keratin sequenced so far has this structural feature of lacking the carboxy-terminal domain. It seems likely that keratin 19 has evolved and been conserved across species for a purpose that depends specifically on this lack of a tail domain. Previous workers have interpreted the in-register extension of the helix as indicating that keratin 19 reflects the more primitive state of an ancestral keratin from which other keratins subsequently evolved, but an α-helical conformation might also be selected as a means of compacting any acquired irrelevant carboxy-terminal peptides out of the way.

A reason for suspecting that keratin 19 is *not* the most primitive of the keratins is its divergence from the sequence of keratin 18 (the type-I keratin expressed in all simple epithelial cells), yet its strong similarity to the keratins of stratified epithelia (which are structurally more elaborate than simple epithelia and arise later in development). This is illustrated in Figure 1, which shows the degree of identity between human keratin 19 and other sequenced type-I keratins, comparing the consensus helical rod domains (Stasiak et al. 1988). Keratin 19 can therefore (at most) only be ancestral to some of the type-I keratins of stratified epithelia. The simple epithelial keratin 18, which is the earliest embryonic type-I keratin, appears to be of a separate and probably older stock.

DISCUSSION
Little is known about the specific functions of the nonhelical domains of intermediate filaments. The "head" (amino-terminal) domain appears to be important for correct filament formation (Kaufmann et al. 1985), if not for the formation of the initial two-chain molecule; this and/or the "tail" (carboxy-terminal) domain may well protrude outside the final filamentous polymer (Geisler et al. 19840. These terminal domains probably modify the properties of the keratins and keratin filaments in a tissue-specific manner. A hypothesis that would link the tissue distribution pattern with the structural absence of a tail domain would be that keratin 19 has been conserved for its ability to act as a "neutral" keratin in terms of differentiation. Keratin 19 is fully competent at polymerization and thus can probably integrate into the transcellular network of keratin filaments and desmosome anchorage junctions, which is fundamental to the structural integrity of an epithelium.

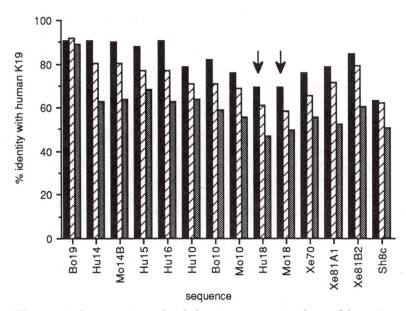

Figure 1 Conservation of rod domain sequences of type-I keratins with respect to human keratin 19, expressed as percentage of amino acids identical with human keratin 19, as far as sequences are available. Consensus helical domain boundaries are taken as TMQN . . . . TYR[X]LLEG[Q/E]; (solid bars) helix 1A; (hatched bars) helix 1B; (stippled bars) helix 2. (Bo19) Bovine homolog of keratin 19 (Bader et al. 1986), (Hu14) human keratin 14 (Hanukoglu and Fuchs 1982); (Mo14B) mouse 50-kD basal-expressed (only 31 amino acids of helix 1A) (Knapp et al. 1987); (Hu15) human keratin 15 (Leube et al. 1988); (Hu16) human keratin 16 (Rosenberg et al. 1988); (Hu10) human keratin 10 (Darmon et al. 1987); (Bo10) bovine keratin VIb, putative homolog of human K10/K11 (Reiger et al. 1985); (Mo10) mouse, putative homolog of human K10 (Steinert et al. 1983); (Hu18) human keratin 18 (Oshima et al. 1986); (Mo18) mouse ENDO B, homolog of human K18 (Singer et al. 1986); (Xe70) *Xenopus laevis* XK70 premetamorphic epidermal keratin (Winkles et al. 1985); (Xe81A1 and Xe81B2) *X. laevis* premetamorphic keratins (Miyatani et al. 1986); (Sh8c) sheep wool keratin 8c (Dowling et al. 1986).

However, it may not fully restrict the cell expressing it to differentiate along either or any available pathway if it lacks the (as yet unidentified) tail-specified differentiation function.

Keratin filaments are always heteropolymers, requiring the presence of both type-I and type-II keratins to form a filament, and the mechanism that coregulates the expression of these keratin pairs is one of the most interesting puzzles in the field. It is known that in many stratified epithelia, the type-II keratin of the differentiation-specific keratin pair is often expressed prior to the type-I partner. Recent data suggest that a single keratin species, unable to polymerize, is not stable in the cytoplasm and may be rapidly degraded (Kulesh and Oshima 1988; X. Lu et al., unpubl.). If keratin 19 is expressed as an intermediate type-I keratin, it may allow delayed synthesis of the specific type-I partner by combining with and stabilizing the type-II keratin synthesized in the basal layer. This would predict that the affinity of keratin-19/type-II complexes would always be lower than the affinity of complexes between coexpressed type-I/type-II keratins, in order to allow the specific type-I keratin to compete away keratin 19 from the filament network once committed synthesis begins; possibly, this is where the tail domains become important in increasing the affinity of complexes between coexpressed pairs.

This model would also predict that type-I keratin expression might be under more stringent tissue-specific regulation than that of the type-II keratins.

A role for keratin 19 as a "switch" keratin could be a mechanism for suspending post-stem-cell-amplifying cells in a flexible or uncommited state of differentiation, which could be a necessary integral control mechanism for maintenance of balanced cell populations across boundaries or within mixed cell populations in complex epithelia. The recognition of a keratin phenotype that marks a cell in a labile state of differentiation may also have clinical implications if such cells are more vulnerable to neoplastic transformation.

REFERENCES

Bader, B.L., T.M. Magin, M. Hatzfeld, and W.W. Franke. 1986. Amino acid sequence and gene organization of cytokeratin no. 19, an exceptional tail-less intermediate filament protein. *EMBO J.* **5:** 1865.

Bartek, J., E.M. Durban, R.C. Hallowes, and J. Taylor-Papadimitriou. 1985. A subclass of luminal epithelial cells in the mammary gland defined by antibodies to cytokeratins. *J. Cell Sci.* **75:** 17.

Bartek, J., J. Bartkova, J. Taylor-Papadimitriou, A. Reijthar, J. Kovarik, Z. Lukas, and A. Vojtesek. 1986. Differential expression of keratin 19 in normal human epithelial tissues revealed by monospecific monoclonal antibodies. *Histochem. J.* **18:** 565.

Darmon, M.Y., A. Sémat, M.C. Darmon, and M. Vasseur. 1987. Sequence of a cDNA encoding human keratin no. 10 selected according to structural homologies of keratins and their tissue-specific expression. *Mol. Biol. Rep.* **12:** 277.

Dowling, L.M., W.G. Crewther, and A.S. Inglis. 1986. The primary structure of component 8c-1, a subunit protein of intermediate filaments in wool keratin. Relationships with proteins from other intermediate filaments. *Biochem. J.* **236:** 695.

Eckert, R.L. 1988. Sequence of the human 40-kDa keratin reveals an unusual structure with very high sequence identity to the corresponding bovine keratin. *Proc. Natl. Acad. Sci.* **85:** 1114.

Franz, J.K. 1987. "Characterization and cloning of cytokeratins from *Xenopus laevis*." Ph.D. thesis, University of Heidelberg, Federal Republic of Germany.

Geisler, N., S. Fischer, J. Vandekerckhove, U. Plessmann, and K. Weber. 1984. Hybrid character of a large neurofilament protein NF-M: Intermediate filament type sequence followed by a long and acidic carboxy-terminal extension. *EMBO J.* **3:** 2701.

Gigi-Leitner, O. and B. Geiger. 1986. Antigenic interrelationship between the 40-kilodalton cytokeratin polypeptide and desmoplakins. *Cell Motil. Cytoskeleton* **6:** 628.

Gigi-Leitner, O., B. Geiger, R. Levy, and B. Czernobilsky. 1986. Cytokeratin expression in sqamous metaplasia of the human uterine cervix. *Differentiation* **31:** 191.

Hanukoglu, I. and E. Fuchs. 1982. The cDNA sequence of a human epidermal keratin: Divergence of sequence but conservation of structure among intermediate filament proteins. *Cell* **31:** 243.

Karsten, U., G. Papsdorf, G. Roloff, P. Stolley, H. Abel, I. Walther, and H. Weiss. 1985. Monoclonal anti-cytokeratin antibody from a hybridoma clone generated by electrofusion. *Eur. J. Cancer Clin. Oncol.* **21:** 733.

Kaufmann, E., K. Weber, and N. Geisler. 1985. Intermediate filament forming ability of desmin derivatives lacking either the aminoterminal 67 or the carboxy-terminal 27 residues. *J. Mol. Biol.* **185:** 733.

Knapp, B., M. Rentrop, J. Schweizer, and H. Winter. 1987. Three cDNA sequences of mouse type I keratins. Cellular localization of the mRNAs in normal and hyperproliferative tissues. *J. Biol. Chem.* **262:** 938.

Kulesh, D.A. and R.G. Oshima. 1988. Cloning of the human K18 gene and its expresison in nonepithelial mouse cells. *Mol. Cell. Biol.* **8:** 1540.

Leube, R.E., B.L. Bader, F.X. Bosch, R. Zimbelmann, T. Achtstätter, and W.W. Franke. 1988. Molecular characterization and expression of the stratification-related cytokeratins 4 and 15. *J. Cell Biol.* **106:** 1249.

Miyatani, S., J.A. Winkles, T.D. Sargent, and I.B. Dawid. 1986. Stage-specific keratins in *Xenopus laevis* embryos and tadpoles: The XK81 gene family. *J. Cell. Biol.* **103:** 1957.

Morgan, P.R., I.M. Leigh, P.E. Purkis, I.D. Gardner, G.N.P. van Muijen, and E.B. Lane. 1987. Site variation in keratin expression in human oral epithelia — An immunocytochemical study of individual keratins. *Epithelia* **1:** 31.

Oshima, R.G., J.L. Milan, and G. Cecena. 1986. Comparison of mouse and human keratin 18: A component of intermediate filaments expressed prior to implantation. *Differentiation* **33:** 61.

Rieger, M., J.L. Jorcano, and W.W. Franke. 1985. Complete sequence of a bovine type I cytokeratin gene: Conserved and variable positions in genes of polypeptides of the same cytokeratin subfamily. *EMBO J.* **4:** 2261.

Rosenberg, M., A. RayChaudury, T.B. Snows, M. LeBeau, and E. Fuchs. 1988. A group of type I keratin genes on human chromosome 17: Characterization and expression. *Mol. Cell. Biol.* **8:** 722.

Singer, P.A., K. Trevor, and R.G. Oshima. 1986. Molecular cloning and characterization of the Endo B cytokeratin expressed in preimplantation mouse embryos. *J. Biol. Chem.* **261:** 538.

Stasiak, P.C. and E.B. Lane. 1987. Sequences of cDNA coding for human keratin 19. *Nucleic Acids Res.* **15:** 10058.

Stasiak, P.C., P.E. Purkis, I.M. Leigh, and E.B. Lane. 1988. Keratin 19: Predicted amino acid sequence and broad tissue distribution suggest it evolved from keratinocyte keratins. *J. Invest. Dermatol.* (in press).

Steinert, P.M., R.H. Rice, D.R. Roop, B.L. Trus, and A.C. Steven. 1983. Complete amino acid sequence of a mouse epidermal keratin subunit and implications for the structure of intermediate filaments. *Nature* **302:** 794.

Sun, T.-T., R. Eichner, A. Schermer, D. Cooper, W.G. Nelson, and R.A. Weiss. 1984. Classification, expression, and possible mechanisms of evolution of mammalian keratins: A unifying model. *Cancer Cells* **1:** 169.

Winkles, J.A., T.D. Sargent, D.A.D. Parry, E. Jonas, and I.B. Dawid. 1985. Developmentally regulated cytokeratin gene in *Xenopus laevis*. *Mol. Cell. Biol.* **5:** 2575.

Wu, Y-J. and J.G. Rheinwald. 1981. A new small 40 kd keratin filament protein made by some cultured human sqamous cell carcinomas. *Cell* **25:** 627.

Intrinsic Differences in Histogenic Potential and Keratin Regulation among Oral Epithelial Cell Types and Dysregulation of Keratin 19 in Oral Premalignant Dysplasia

J.G. Rheinwald,[1,2] K. Lindberg,[1,3] M.E. Brown,[1] and T.M. O'Connell[1]

[1]Division of Cell Growth and Regulation
Dana-Farber Cancer Institute, Boston, Massachusetts 02115

[2]Department of Cellular and Molecular Physiology
Harvard Medical School, Boston, Massachusetts 02115

[3]Department of Oral Pathology and Oral Medicine
Harvard School of Dental Medicine,
Boston, Massachusetts 02115

The oral cavity is lined by stratified squamous epithelium. This epithelium is regionally variable in the program of terminal differentiation followed by the keratinocytes after they leave the basal layer and move upward to form the multilayered tissue. The areas covered by so-called lining mucosa (i.e., bucca, floor of mouth, underside of tongue, and soft palate) display a type of differentiation referrred to as nonkeratinization, in that the outermost cells retain their nuclei and do not become extremely flattened. In contrast, the areas covered by so-called masticatory mucosa (i.e., gingiva, hard palate, and retromolar pads) usually display a type of differentiation referred to as parakeratinization, in that the outermost cells retain their nuclei but become very flat, forming a stratum corneum. This type of differentiation resembles, but is not identical to, the orthokeratinization of the epidermis, in which cells synthesize keratohyalin granules and membrane-coating granules before losing their nuclei and forming a stratum corneum.

Stratified squamous epithelial differentiation is associated with the expression of specialized keratin proteins in the suprabasal cells. The keratins, or cytokeratins, are one of the five distinctive families of cytoplasmic intermediate filament proteins. Keratin filaments are formed from tetrameric building blocks composed of two different types of protein subunits from among a family of about 25 members of 40-67 kD, each of which appears to be encoded by a separate gene (Moll et al. 1982; Fuchs et al. 1987). From two to ten different keratins are expressed by each epithelial cell type (Moll et al. 1982; Tseng et al. 1982; Wu et al. 1982). The basal cells of all stratified squamous epithelia express the K5/K14 keratin pair, and cells retain these keratins but no longer synthesize them after they move upward and terminally differentiate (Tyner and Fuchs 1986). Orthokeratinized epithelia express the K1/K10 keratin pair in the suprabasal cells, nonkeratinized epithelia such as oral lining mucosa express the K4/K13 pair suprabasally, and parakeratinized epithelia such as oral masticatory mucosa express both pairs, not necessarily in the same suprabasal cell (Cooper et al. 1985; Ouhayoun et al. 1985; Morgan et al. 1987).

A number of years ago, our studies of keratin expression in malignant keratinocytes (squamous carcinoma cells [SCC]) originating from these tissues had disclosed abnormally high K19 expression in some, but not all, SCC lines in culture (Wu and Rheinwald 1981). This originally suggested to us that immunohistochemical staining for K19 may be of some diagnostic value for this type of cancer, but the discovery that some normal epithelial cell types express K19 at high levels (Moll et al. 1982; Tseng et al. 1982; Wu et al. 1982) distracted us from pursuing a possible association between K19 and malignant transformation in keratinocytes. Recently, however, as part of a project to understand the basis of histologic diversity in the oral epithelium, we decided to reexamine K19 expression as a function of regional and malignant change.

We used cell culture and transplantation methods to investigate the extent to which intrinsic, permanent characteristics of the differentiated state of oral epithelial cells, as opposed to instructive influences from the local connective tissue, are responsible for the regional specialization seen in the oral epithelia. We cultured cells from both nonkeratinized and parakeratinized regions using the 3T3 feeder layer system (Rheinwald and Green 1975; Allen-Hoffmann and Rheinwald 1984 and references therein). Cells from nonkeratinized regions (bucca, floor of mouth, ventral tongue, and soft palate) formed slightly less stratified colonies than did cells cultured from keratinized regions (gingiva and hard palate). Soft palatal epithelial cells could be distinguished from cells cultured from all other regions by their whorling colony morphology and absence of stratification. Cells cultured from all sites synthesized keratins K5, K6, K14, K16, and K17, and those cultured from nonkeratinized regions also expressed variable amounts of K13 and K19. In addition to these seven keratins, soft palatal cells also expressed the simple epithelial keratins, K7, K8, and K18.

Using a grafting technique described recently by Barrandon et al. (1988), we determined the type of differentiation and pattern of keratins that cells cultured from each site would express when returned to an in vivo environment, lacking any potential regional signals or cues that might induce a particular pathway of differentiation (K. Lindberg and J. Rheinwald, in prep.). Confluent cultures of cells that had undergone from 15 to 30 divisions in vitro were released as an intact sheet and grafted against the underside of the dermis of a *nude* mouse. One week after grafting, keratinocytes that had been cultured from a biopsy taken from the floor of the mouth formed a nonkeratinized epithelium and expressed K19 (disclosed by the A53-B/A2 antibody; Karsten et al. 1985) in all basal cells and expressed K13 (disclosed by the AE8 antibody; Dhouailly et al. 1989) in all suprabasal cells, identical to the native epithelium (Fig. 1). Keratinocytes cultured from the gingiva formed a mostly parakeratinized but partly nonkeratinized epithelium in which most of the basal cells were K19-negative and all the suprabasal cells were K13-positive and K1/K10-negative (the latter assessed by staining with the antibody AE2; Woodcock-Mitchell et al. 1982). Keratinocytes cultured from epidermis underwent orthokeratinization in the grafts, complete with keratohyalin granules, suprabasal K1/K10 expression, and no K13 expression.

These results show that regional variation of stratified squamous epithelial differentiation in the oral mucosa is based on intrinsic characteristics of the keratinocyte subtype that forms the epithelium in each region. The incompletely parakeratinized epithelium formed by cultured gingival keratinocytes suggests that although this keratinocyte subtype is indeed intrinsically different from the lining mucosal keratinocyte, expression of the full differentiation potential of oral parakeratinizing epithelial cells may require specific environmental factors not provided by the experimental graft bed.

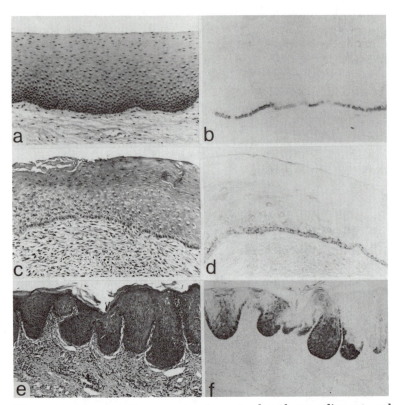

Figure 1 Keratin 19 expression in normal and premalignant oral lining mucosal epithelium. (*a,c,e*) Hematoxylin/eosin-stained sections; (*b,d,f*) avidin-biotin-peroxidase immunostaining for keratin 19 of nearby sections of the same specimens. (*a,b*) Normal human floor of mouth epithelium; (*c,d*) stratified epithelium formed by transplanting a confluent sheet of cultured normal human floor of mouth keratinocytes (strain OKF4) to the underside of the dermis of an athymic *nude* mouse, 1 week after grafting; (*e,f*) premalignant lesion exhibiting moderate-to-severe dysplasia from the floor of mouth. Note that expression of keratin 19 restricted to cells in the basal layer of nonkeratinized stratified squamous epithelia is an intrinsic property of the cells and that retention of keratin 19 in suprabasal cells accompanies premalignant dysplasia in such tissues.

We next studied the expression of keratin K19 in oral lesions exhibiting a range of histopathologic changes that are thought to precede SCC. Formalin-fixed, parafffin-embedded sections from pathology files of Boston-area hospitals were pretreated with pronase (Battifora and Kopinski 1986) and stained with the K19-specific A53-B/A2 antibody (Karsten et al.

1985) (obtained as antibody K_s-19.1 from Progen, Heidelberg, or ICN Biomedicals, Lisle, Illinois). K19 antigenicity was blocked by formalin fixation, but we found that the antigen recognized by this antibody was exposed by protease treatment in about half the cases examined. To ensure that epithelia that did not stain with the antibody were truly K19-negative, we only included data from samples that showed staining of normal lining mucosal epithelial basal cells or normal salivary duct epithelial cells in the same section, thus providing an internal positive control against irreversible antigen damage from the formalin.

As we have reported recently (Lindberg and Rheinwald 1989), nonkeratinized mucosa, whether normal or benign hyperplastic, stained for K19 in the basal cell layer alone. There was no detectable K19 in any cells of parakeratinized mucosa, whether the tissue specimen was normal or benign hyperplastic. All lesions from any oral site that exhibited atypia diagnosed from hematoxylin/eosin-stained sections as moderate-to-severe dysplasia or carcinoma in situ, whether keratinized or not, stained strongly for K19 in the basal and the suprabasal cell layers. The number of suprabasal cell layers that were K19-positive correlated with the level in the epithelium to which dysplasia persisted. Interestingly, about half the specimens of fully invasive oral SCC examined were K19-negative, indicating that genetic or epigenetic changes occurring at later stages of neoplastic progression frequently result in substantial derangement of the keratin regulation system characteristic of the epithelial cell type from which the cancer originated. In this connection, we found that the pattern of keratins synthesized in culture by ten squamous carcinomas that had arisen from the floor of mouth, ventral tongue, soft palate, and epidermis did not resemble that of normal cells from the respective sites (K. Lindberg and J.G. Rheinwald, in prep.).

Suprabasal K19 tended to occur in epithelial lesions in which expression of the terminal differentiation protein involucrin was delayed or absent. Thus, K19 expression may be linked to the retention of division potential or to a state uncommitted to terminal differentiation. Suprabasal K19 staining is clearly correlated with premalignant change in oral epithelium and therefore promises to be a useful tool in oral histopathological diagnosis. As basal-cell-restricted K19 expression has been found in normal esophageal and exocervical epithelium (Dixon and Stanley 1984; Bosch et al. 1988), examination of lesions of these tissues is warranted to determine whether a similar association between suprabasal K19 and premalignancy is present.

ACKNOWLEDGMENTS

This research was supported by grants from the National Cancer Institute to J.G.R. J.G.R. was the recipient of a faculty research award from the American Cancer Society. K.L. was supported by a training grant from the National Institutes of Health to the Department of Oral Pathology and Oral Medicine, Harvard School of Dental Medicine.

REFERENCES

Allen-Hoffmann, B.L. and J.G. Rheinwald. 1984. Polycyclic aromatic hydrocarbon mutagenesis of human epidermal keratinocytes in culture. *Proc. Natl. Acad. Sci.* **81:** 7802.

Barrandon, Y., V. Li, and H. Green. 1988. New techniques for the grafting of cultured human epidermal cells onto athymic animals. *J. Invest. Dermatol.* **91:** 315.

Battifora, H. and M. Kopinski. 1986. The influence of protease digestion and duration of fixation on the immunostaining of keratins. A comparison of formalin and ethanol fixation. *J. Histochem. Cytochem.* **34:** 1095.

Bosch, F.X., R.E. Leube, T. Achstatter, R. Moll, and W.W. Franke. 1988. Expression of simple epithelial type cytokeratins in stratified epithelia as detected by immunolocalization and hybridization in situ. *J. Cell Biol.* **106:** 1635.

Cooper, D., A. Schermer, and T.-T. Sun. 1985. Classification of human epithelia and their neoplasms using monoclonal antibodies to keratins: Strategies, applications, and limitations. *Lab. Invest.* **52:** 243.

Dixon, I.S. and M.A. Stanley. 1984. Immunofluorescent studies of human cervical epithelia *in vivo* and *in vitro* using antibodies against specific keratin components. *Mol. Biol. Med.* **2:** 37.

Dhouailly, D., C. Xu, M. Manabe, and T.-T. Sun. 1989. Expression of hair-related keratins in soft epithelia: Subpopulation of human and mouse dorsal tongue keratinocytes express keratin markers for hair, skin, and esophageal types of differentiation. *Exp. Cell Res.* (in press).

Fuchs, E., A.L. Tyner, G.J. Giudice, D. Marchuk, A. RayChaudhury, and N. Rosenberg. 1987. The human keratin genes and their differentiated expression. *Curr. Top. Dev. Biol.* **22:** 5.

Karsten, U., G. Papsdorf, G. Roloff, P. Stolley, H. Abel, I. Walther, and H. Weiss. 1985. Monoclonal anti-cytokeratin antibody from a hybridoma clone generated by electrofusion. *Eur. J. Cancer Clin. Oncol.* **21:** 733.

Lindberg, K. and J.G. Rheinwald. 1989. Suprabasal 40kd (K19) expression as an immunohistological marker of premalignancy in oral epithelium. *Am. J. Pathol.* **134:** (in press).

Moll, R., W.W. Franke, D.L. Schiller, B. Geiger, and R. Krepler. 1982.

The catalog of human cytokeratins: Patterns of expression in normal epithelia, tumors, and cultured cells. *Cell* **31**: 11.

Morgan, P.R., I.M. Leigh, P.E. Purkis, I.D. Gardner, G.N.P. van Muijen, and E.B. Lane. 1987. Site variation in keratin expression in human oral epithelia — An immunocytochemical study of individual keratins. *Epithelia* **1**: 31.

Ouhayoun, J.-P., F. Gosselin, N. Forest, S. Winter, and W.W. Franke. 1985. Cytokeratin patterns of human oral epithelia: Differences in cytokeratin synthesis in gingival epithelium and the adjacent alveolar mucosa. *Differentiation* **30**: 123.

Rheinwald, J.G. and H. Green. 1975. Serial cultivation of strains of human epidermal keratinocytes: The formation of keratinizing colonies from single cells. *Cell* **6**: 331.

Tseng, S.C.G., M.J. Jarvinen, W.G. Nelson, J.-W. Huang, J. Woodcock-Mitchell, and T.-T. Sun. 1982. Correlation of specific keratins with different types of epithelial differentiation: Monoclonal antibody studies. *Cell* **30**: 361.

Tyner, A.L. and E. Fuchs. 1986. Evidence for post-transcriptional regulation of the keratins expressed during hyperproliferation and malignant transformation in human epidermis. *J. Cell Biol.* **103**: 1945.

Woodcock-Mitchell, J., R. Eichner, W.G. Nelson, and T.-T. Sun. 1982. Immunolocalization of keratin polypeptides in human epidermis using monoclonal antibodies. *J. Cell Biol.* **95**: 580.

Wu, J.-J. and J.G. Rheinwald. 1981. A new small (40kd) keratin filament protein made by some cultured human squamous cell carcinomas. *Cell* **25**: 627.

Wu, Y.-J., L.M. Parker, N.E. Binder, M.A. Beckett, J.H. Sinard, C.T. Griffiths, and J.G. Rheinwald. 1982. The mesothelial keratins: A new family of cytoskeletal proteins identified in cultured mesothelial cells and nonkeratinizing epithelia. *Cell* **31**: 693.

The Use of Specific Keratin Antisera and Nucleic Acid Probes to Monitor Different Stages of Skin Carcinogenesis

D.R. Roop,[1] T. Mehrel, T.M. Krieg,[2] H. Nakazawa, C.K. Cheng, and S.H. Yuspa

Laboratory of Cellular Carcinogenesis and Tumor Promotion
Division of Cancer Etiology, National Cancer Institute
Bethesda, Maryland 20892

The process of terminal differentiation is highly regulated in mouse epidermis and occurs in stages. Terminal differentiation begins with the migration of cells from the basal layer, continues with the progression of cells through the spinous and granular layers, and ends with the deposition of the mature epidermal cells (squames) in the stratum corneum. The commitment to enter the differentiation program appears to occur postmitotically, as DNA synthesis and cell division are restricted to the basal layer. Changes in keratin gene expression occur during epidermal differentiation (Roop et al. 1988). Keratins K5 and K14 are major products of basal epidermal cells. K5 is a member of the type-II intermediate filament (IF) subclass, and K14 is a member of the type-I IF subclass (Steinert and Roop 1988). The presence of both K5 and K14 is required for keratin filament formation, and these filaments, together with microtubules (tubulin) and microfilaments (actin), form the cytoskeleton of epidermal cells. One of the earliest changes associated with the commitment to differentiation and migration into the spinous layer is induction of another differentiation-specific pair of keratins: K1 (type II) and K10 (type I). IFs containing K1 and K10 replace those containing K5 and K14 as the major products of cells in the spinous and granular layer.

Several laboratories have reported changes in keratin expression in mouse tumors produced in the skin carcinogenesis

Present addresses: [1]Departments of Cell Biology and Dermatology, Baylor College of Medicine, Houston, Texas 77030; [2]Dermatologische Klinik and Poliklinik, Der Ludwig-Maximilians-Universitaet, Munich, Federal Republic of Germany.

model (Nelson and Slaga 1982; Winter and Schweizer 1983; Toftgard et al. 1985). In addition to keratins K5, K14, K1, and K10 expressed in normal mouse epidermis, papillomas express keratins K6 and K16 (Nakazawa et al. 1986; Knapp et al. 1987), which are expressed in skin and other tissues under conditions of hyperproliferation (Moll et al. 1984; Weiss et al. 1984). There is a dramatic decrease in expression of K1 and K10 in malignant skin tumors, as revealed by studies at the mRNA (Toftgard et al. 1985) and protein (Nelson and Slaga 1982; Winter and Schweizer 1983) levels.

Sensitive methods to monitor keratin gene expression would be very useful in skin carcinogenesis studies. Such methods might allow the detection of early changes, which precede the appearance of benign tumors, and the recognition of malignant conversion at a preclinical stage. Therefore, we initiated a project to isolate genes encoding keratins expressed at different differentiation states. This approach allowed us to isolate and sequence all of the major keratins expressed in mouse epidermis, including keratins K5 and K14, expressed predominantly in proliferating basal cells (Steinert et al. 1984; Roop et al. 1985), and keratins K1 and K10, expressed predominantly in differentiated epidermal cells (Steinert et al. 1983, 1985). In addition, we isolated a cDNA clone for keratin K6, which is expressed under hyperproliferative conditions such as cell culture but not in normal epidermis (Nakazawa et al. 1986).

Sequence analysis of these cloned cDNAs has revealed unique amino acids at the carboxyl terminus of individual keratin proteins (Steinert et al. 1983, 1984, 1985; Krieg et al. 1985). Synthetic peptides corresponding to these sequences have been used to elicit monospecific antibodies (Roop et al. 1984, 1985). These antibodies have been useful reagents to study the specific expression of individual keratin proteins within particular cell types (Roop et al. 1987, 1988). In addition, the sequence information has enabled us to produce specific nucleic acid probes for the analysis of transcriptional activity by in situ hybridization (Roop et al. 1986, 1988). These specific reagents have been used to monitor different stages of skin carcinogenesis.

Keratin Expression during Stages of Skin Carcinogenesis

Early Events Preceding the Appearance of Benign Lesions
The gene encoding keratin K6 is normally never expressed in the epidermis (Nakazawa et al. 1986). However, its expression

is quickly triggered when changes in the proliferative status of epidermal cells occur. These changes can be induced experimentally by topical application of TPA or tape stripping. All benign and malignant epidermal tumors examined to date express K6. We suspect that expression of the K6 gene occurs very early in skin carcinogenesis. The ability to detect K6 may allow the identification of altered foci before they become apparent as a benign lesion. Experimentally, this would facilitate the identification of genetic changes that occur very early during initiation-promotion protocols.

Early Events Associated with Malignant Conversion

Three independent laboratories have documented the absence of the differentiation-specific keratins (K1 and K10) in malignant mouse skin tumors, resulting from initiation-promotion protocols (Nelson and Slaga 1982; Winter and Schweizer 1983; Toftgard et al. 1985). We have recently used antibodies specific for these keratins to demonstrate that these changes occur early during conversion (Roop et al. 1988). Our observations have been confirmed independently by Aldaz et al. (1988). These investigators have also correlated these changes in keratin expression with the expression of glutamyltransferase, which has been shown previously to occur in malignant but not benign tumors (Klein-Szanto et al. 1983), and changes in chromosomal status, which appear to occur progressively during skin carcinogenesis (Aldaz et al. 1987). Therefore, the loss of keratins K1 and K10 appears to be an early negative marker for conversion from benign to malignant status.

In addition to these keratins serving as negative markers for conversion, keratin K13 has recently been shown to be a potential positive marker for conversion (Nischt et al. 1988). These observations resulted from a collaboration between our laboratory and that of J. Schweizer. K13 is normally expressed in the suprabasal layers of internally stratifying epithelia. It is not expressed in normal epidermis, nor is it expressed under hyperproliferative conditions induced in vivo or in vitro. However, a combination of immunological analysis, employing a specific antiserum produced against a unique synthetic peptide, and in situ hybridization analysis, using a specific nucleic acid probe, revealed that K13 was expressed in carcinomas resulting from initiation-promotion protocols. In addition, the number of papillomas expressing K13 was found to increase with the time of promotion. Additional experiments will be re-

117

quired to determine whether there is a correlation between the loss of keratin K1 and K10 and the appearance of K13. Nevertheless, the appearance of K13 may provide a positive marker for malignant conversion.

The availability of markers to detect malignant conversion at stages prior to gross or histological examination would be of particular importance in experimental studies. Experiments designed to determine the potency of genotoxic agents undoubtedly underestimate their potency because animals usually die as a result of the first or second malignant tumor. The ability to screen for early signs of conversion would permit the assessment of the conversion state of all tumors at the time of death and provide a more accurate estimate of the potency of genotoxic agents. In addition to this application, the detection of conversion at an early stage may assist in the identification of primary genetic events required for conversion.

Application to the Diagnosis of Human Skin Cancer
Insufficient data are currently available to determine how useful these observations will be in the study and diagnosis of human skin cancers. The presence of K6 has been reported in human skin tumors (Moll et al. 1984; Weiss et al. 1984). However, there are no reports correlating the expression of K6 with early stages of carcinogenesis. Human squamous cell carcinomas generally have reduced levels of differentiation-specific keratins (Moll et al. 1982, 1984; Winter et al. 1983; Nelson et al. 1984; Huszar et al. 1986). However, a large percentage have minor, but significant, amounts of these proteins (Moll et al. 1984; Huszar et al. 1986). K13 expression has not been observed in human skin cancers. Thus, at the present time, these changes in keratin expression are only suitable for monitoring skin carcinogenesis in the mouse model. The development of antisera and nucleic acid probes to specifically detect human keratins is required to determine whether these observations will eventually be useful in the diagnosis of human skin cancer.

REFERENCES
Aldaz, C.M., C.J. Conti, A.J.P. Klein-Szanto, and T.J. Slaga. 1987. Progressive dysplasia and aneuploidy are hallmarks of mouse skin papillomas: Relevance to malignancy. *Proc. Natl. Acad. Sci.* **84:** 2029.
Aldaz, C.M., C.J. Conti, F. Larcher, D. Trono, D.R. Roop, J. Chesner, T. Whitehead, and T.J. Slaga. 1988. Sequential development of aneuploidy, keratin modification, and γ-glutamyltransferase expression in mouse skin papillomas. *Cancer Res.* **48:** 3253.

Huszar, M., O. Gigi-Leitner, R. Moll, W.W. Franke, and B. Geiger. 1986. Monoclonal antibodies to various acidic (type I) cytokeratins of stratified epithelia. *Differentiation* **31**: 141.

Klein-Szanto, A.J.P., K.G. Nelson, Y. Shah, and T.J. Slaga. 1983. Simultaneous appearance of keratin modifications and γ-glutamyltransferase activity as indicators of tumor progression in mouse skin papillomas. *J. Natl. Cancer Inst.* **70**: 161.

Knapp, B., M. Rentrop, J. Schweizer, and H. Winter. 1987. Three cDNA sequences of mouse type I keratins: Cellular localization of the mRNAs in normal and hyperproliferative tissues. *J. Biol. Chem.* **262**: 938.

Kreig, T.M., M.P. Schafer, C.K. Cheng, D. Filpula, P. Flaherty, P.M. Steinert, and D.R. Roop. 1985. Organization of a type I keratin gene: Evidence for evolution of intermediate filaments from a common ancestral gene. *J. Biol. Chem.* **260**: 5867.

Moll, R., I. Moll, and W.W. Franke. 1984. Differences in expression of cytokeratin polypeptides in various epithelial skin tumors. *Arch. Dermatol. Res.* **276**: 349.

Moll, R., W.W. Franke, D.L. Schiller, B. Geiger, and R. Krepler. 1982. The catalog of human cytokeratins: Patterns of expression in normal epithelia, tumors and cultured cells. *Cell* **31**: 11.

Nakazawa, H., T. Mehrel, C.K. Cheng, S.H. Yuspa, and D.R. Roop. 1986. Isolation of cDNA clone encoding a keratin expressed under hyperproliferative conditions. *J. Cell Biol.* **103**: 561a.

Nelson, K.G. and T.J. Slaga. 1982. Keratin modifications in epidermis, papillomas, and carcinomas during two-stage carcinogenesis in the SENCAR mouse. *Cancer Res.* **42**: 4176.

Nelson, W.G., H. Battifora, H. Santana, and T.T. Sun. 1984. Specific keratins as molecular markers for neoplasms with a stratified epithelial origin. *Cancer Res.* **44**: 1600.

Nischt, R., D.R. Roop, T. Mehrel, S.H. Yuspa, M. Rentrop, H. Winter, and J. Schweizer. 1988. Aberrant expression during two stage mouse skin carcinogenesis of a type I 47 kd keratin, k13, normally associated with terminal differentiation of internal stratified epithelia. *Mol. Carcinog.* **1**: 96.

Roop, D.R., H. Huitfeldt, A. Kilkenny, and S.H. Yuspa. 1987. Regulated expression of differentiation-associated keratins in cultured epidermal cells detected by monospecific antibodies to unique peptides of mouse epidermal keratins. *Differentiation* **35**: 143.

Roop, D.R., T.M. Krieg, T. Mehrel, C.K. Cheng, and S.H. Yuspa. 1988. Transcriptional control of high molecular weight keratin gene expression in multistage skin carcinogenesis. *Cancer Res.* **48**: 3245.

Roop, D.R., C.K. Cheng, R. Toftgard, J.R. Stanley, P.M. Steinert, and S.H. Yuspa. 1985. The use of cDNA clones and monospecific antibodies as probes to monitor keratin gene expression. *Ann. N.Y. Acad. Sci.* **455**: 426.

Roop, D.R., C.K. Cheng, L. Titterington, C.A. Meyers, J.R. Stanley, P.M. Steinert, and S.H. Yuspa. 1984. Synthetic peptides corresponding to keratin subunits elicit highly specific antibodies. *J. Biol. Chem.* **259**: 8037.

Roop, D.R., D.R. Lowy, P.E. Tambourin, J. Strickand, J.R. Harper, M. Balaschak, E.F. Spangler, and S.H. Yuspa. 1986. An activated

Harvey *ras* oncogene produces benign tumors on mouse epidermis. *Nature* **323:** 822.

Steinert, P.M. and D.R. Roop. 1988. Molecular and cellular biology of intermediate filaments. *Annu. Rev. Biochem.* **57:** 593.

Steinert, P.M., R.H. Rice, D.R. Roop, B.L. Trus, and A.C. Steven. 1983. Complete amino acid sequence of a mouse epidermal keratin subunit: Implications for the structure of intermediate filaments. *Nature* **302:** 794.

Steinert, P.M., D.A.D. Parry, W.W. Idler, L.D. Johnson, A.C. Steven, and D.R. Roop. 1985. Amino acid sequences of mouse and human epidermal type II keratins of M_r 67,000 provide a systematic basis for the structural and functional diversity of the end domains of keratin intermediate filament subunits. *J. Biol. Chem.* **260:** 7142.

Steinert, P.M., D.A.D. Parry, E.L. Racoosin, W.W. Idler, A.C. Steven, B.L. Trus, and D.R. Roop. 1984. The complete cDNA and deduced amino acid sequence of a type II mouse epidermal keratin of 60,000 Da: Analysis of sequence differences between type I and type II keratins. *Proc. Natl. Acad. Sci.* **81:** 5709.

Toftgard, R., S.H. Yuspa, and D.R. Roop. 1985. Keratin gene expression in mouse skin tumors and in mouse skin treated with TPA. *Cancer Res.* **45:** 5845.

Weiss, R.A., R.A. Eichner, and T.-T. Sun. 1984. Monoclonal antibody analysis of keratin expression in epidermal diseases: A 48- and 56-kilodalton keratin as molecular markers for hyperproliferative keratinocytes. *J. Cell Biol.* **98:** 1397.

Winter, H. and J. Schweizer. 1983. Keratin synthesis in normal mouse epithelia and in squamous cell carcinomas: Evidence in tumors for masked mRNA species coding for high molecular weight kera-tin polypeptides. *Proc. Natl. Acad. Sci.* **80:** 6480.

Winter, H., J. Schweizer, and K. Goerttler. 1983. Keratin polypeptide composition as a biochemical tool for the discrimination of benign and malignant epithelial lesions in man. *Arch. Dermatol. Res.* **275:** 27.

Pathways of Keratinocyte Differentiation

T.-T. Sun

Epithelial Biology Unit
Departments of Dermatology and Pharmacology
New York University Medical School
New York, New York 10016

The keratinocyte is the major cell type found in epidermis, corneal epithelium, esophageal epithelium, exocervical epithelium, and other stratified squamous epithelia. Although keratinocytes of all these epithelia share some common features such as the synthesis of large quantities of keratins (which account for ~30% of their total proteins), data from cell culture and transplantation experiments indicate that keratinocytes of skin, cornea, and esophagus are intrinsically divergent, as evidenced by their capability of expressing different sets of keratins, even under identical cell cultures, as well as in vivo environments (Doran et al. 1980). As far as the expression of keratins within a given stratified epithelium is concerned, we and other investigators have shown that basal cells of several normal stratified epithelia make predominantly the same pair of basic K5 (58K) and acidic K14 (50K) keratins, whereas their suprabasal cells are characterized by additional keratin pairs that are somewhat tissue-specific (Woodcock-Mitchell et al. 1982; Skerrow and Skerrow 1983; Schweizer et al. 1984; Rentrop et al. 1986; Schermer et al. 1986; Lersch and Fuchs 1988; Leube et al. 1988; Stoler et al. 1988). These suprabasally expressed, differentiation-related keratin pairs include K1–2(65–67K)/K10(56.5K), K3(64K)/K12(55K), and K4(59K)/K13(51K) pairs that are found in three prototypic epithelia, i.e., the epidermis, corneal epithelium, and esophageal epithelium, respectively (Sun et al. 1984).

The synthesis of these suprabasal keratin pairs appears to be subject to stringent control, as they tend to diminish under hyperproliferative conditions. When this occurs, suprabasal cells, regardless of their tissue origin, make a common keratin pair K6(56K)/K16–17(46–48K) (Nelson and Sun 1983; Schermer et al. 1986; Stoler et al. 1988). These and other data on the common and cell-type-specific expression of several keratin pairs in the basal versus suprabasal compartments of various stratified squamous epithelia have implications on the pathways of keratinocyte differentiation. In this paper, I briefly describe a hypothesis, illustrated in two cartoons (Galvin et al. 1988), regarding our current understanding of these differentiation pathways.

Reciprocal Expression of Differentiation and Hyperproliferation Markers—A Binary Decision Hypothesis

Our earlier analyses of keratins in various epidermal diseases indicate that the level of K1–2/K10 keratins correlated reasonably well with the degree of morphological keratinization (Weiss et al. 1984). Our data also indicated that the K6/K16 keratins are expressed in many hyperproliferative diseases at a level inversely proportional to that of the keratinization markers (Weiss et al. 1984). We have recently extended this observation to cultured rabbit corneal epithelial cells by [^{35}S]methionine incorporation (A. Schermer et al., in prep.). Taken together, the data suggest a control mechanism by which the total level of differentiation and hyperproliferative markers in a stratified epithelium is kept roughly constant. This can be easily explained if one hypothesizes that in suprabasal cells, the synthesis of the differentiation marker pair and the K6/K16 hyperproliferative pair utilizes a common set or partially overlapping sets of, for example, transcription factors and is therefore mutually exclusive.

In deciding which keratin pair to make, keratinocytes most likely respond to various growth factors and extracellular matrix molecules. Circumstantial evidence is also available that the decisions are not irreversible because even upper cells appear to be capable of responding to environmental cues, such as wounding or the removal of vitamin A in culture medium (Tseng et al. 1984; Eichner et al. 1987). This hypothesis is illustrated in a cartoon in Figure 1. A similar diagram can be made for corneal and esophageal epithelial cells simply by changing the label (and keratin markers) of the upper pathway to a corneal or esophageal type of differentiation. It should be emphasized that this model does not exclude the possiblity that the two types of keratin markers (on both protein and mRNA levels) coexist in the same cell. The value of this hypothesis lies in the fact that (1) it can account for the reciprocal expres-

122

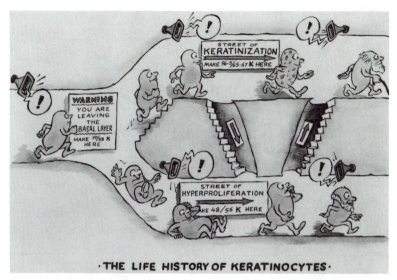

·THE LIFE HISTORY OF KERATINOCYTES·

Figure 1 A cartoon illustrating a hypothesis on epidermal differentiation emphasizing binary decision making when cells enter the suprabasal layer. Cells make such a decision in responding to the sum of external signals (loudspeakers in cartoon). By changing the label (and keratin markers) of the upper pathway, this hypothesis can also be applied to corneal and esophageal epithelium (see text for details; see also Fig. 2). (Reprinted, with permission, from Galvin et al. 1988.)

sion of keratin markers for hyperproliferation and differentiation (Weiss et al. 1984; Schermer et al. 1986), (2) it explains the continuous spectrum of morphological and keratin changes observed in epidermal and other keratinocyte diseases (Weiss et al. 1984), (3) it suggests that upper cells in, for example, psoriatic epidermis undergo an "alternative" pathway of terminal differentiation, rather than "incomplete keratinization" (Galvin et al. 1988; see also Mansbridge et al. 1984), and (4) it suggests a novel mechanism of binary decision making in the expression of suprabasal keratins.

Keratinocyte Differentiation—An Integrated View
Corneal, skin, and esophageal epithelia are all stratified squamous epithelia composed mainly of keratinocytes. Although they are morphologically distinct, they share many common features as far as keratin expression is concerned. I have synthesized these common features, as well as some distinctiveness, into another cartoon (Fig. 2):

123

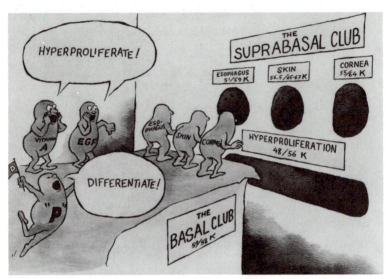

Figure 2 A cartoon illustrating the importance of both extrinsic factors (the cheerleaders) and intrinsic specialization (leg differentiation) in keratinocyte differentiation (see text for details). (Reprinted, with permission, from Galvin et al. 1988.)

1. The basal cells of all three epithelia make the K5/K14–15 keratins (the basal club in Fig. 2).
2. In a permissive environment, the suprabasal cells of these three epithelia make tissue-specific keratin pairs. These pairs are the K1–2/K10, K3/K12, and K4/K13 keratins for the skin, corneal, and esophageal epithelia, respectively (the three upper "tunnels"). However, it should be emphasized that such markers are not truly tissue-specific. For example, during vitamin A deficiency, conjunctival, corneal, and esophageal epithelia can be induced to express small amounts of skin-type markers (Fuchs and Green 1981; Tseng et al. 1984; Cooper et al. 1985; thus, the open space between the basal and suprabasal "clubs" to indicate this potential flexibility).
3. Under hyperplastic conditions, all three epithelia lose their respective differentiation markers and instead make the same K6/K16–17 keratins (Sun and Green 1977; Doran et al. 1980; Nelson and Sun 1983; thus, the shared lower tunnel).
4. When cultured rabbit skin, corneal, and esophageal epi-

thelial cells are placed in identical subcutaneous sites in athymic mice, each cell type regains its in vivo phenotype both in morphology and in keratin pattern (Doran et al. 1980). This illustrates the importance of intrinsic divergence (cell specialization) in regulating epithelial differentiation (represented in the diagram by the "differentiation" between the strength of the right and left "legs," which determine the direction of the "jump" and thus the preferred "upper tunnel" or pathway of differentiation). That all epithelia can differentiate quite normally in the same subcutaneous site also demonstrates that site-specific mesenchymal instruction probably does not play a major role in normal keratinocyte differentiation (Doran et al. 1980).

5. Upon leaving the basal layer, each cell will make a choice of whether to express differentiation markers or hyperproliferation markers. This decision is largely influenced by the sum of all extrinsic signals (the "cheerleaders"). As mentioned earlier, these signals include serum growth factors and vitamin A (which in general stimulate cell growth; Fuchs and Green 1981; Eichner et al. 1984) and the normal in vivo environment (which encourages normal differentiation, labeled "p" for permissiveness to reflect our ignorance of its exact nature; Doran et al. 1980). Additional experiments are needed to test the validity of these working hypotheses by, for example, studying the molecular mechanisms of paired keratin expression and the reciprocal expression of hyperproliferation- and differentiation-related keratin markers.

REFERENCES

Cooper, D., A. Schermer, and T.-T. Sun. 1985. Classification of human epithelia and their neoplasms using monoclonal antikeratin antibodies: Strategies, applications and limitations. *Lab. Invest.* **52:** 243.

Doran, T.I., A. Vidrich, and T.-T. Sun. 1980. Intrinsic and extrinsic regulation of the differentiation of skin, corneal and esophageal epithelial cells. *Cell* **22:** 17.

Eichner, R., P. Bonitz, and T.-T. Sun. 1984. Classification of epidermal keratins according to their immunoreactivity, isoelectric point, and mode of expression. *J. Cell Biol.* **98:** 1388.

Eichner, R., R.A. Weiss, A. Torres, and T.-T. Sun. 1987. Keratin expression in psoriatic and tape-stripping human epidermis. In *Psoriasis: Proceedings of the 4th International Symposium* (ed. E.M. Farber et al.), p. 36. Elsevier, New York.

Fuchs, E. and H. Green. 1981. Regulation of terminal differentiation of cultured human keratinocytes by vitamin A. *Cell* **25:** 617.

Galvin, S., C. Loomis, M. Manabe, D. Dhouailly, and T.-T. Sun. 1988. The major pathways of keratinocyte differentiation as defined by keratin expression: An overview. *Adv. Dermatol.* **4**: 277.

Lersch, R. and E. Fuchs. 1988. Sequence and expression of a type II keratin, K5, in human epidermal cells. *Mol. Cell. Biol.* **8**: 486.

Leube, R.E., L.B. Bader, F.X. Bosch, R. Zimbelmann, T. Achtstaetter, and W.W. Franke. 1988. Molecular characterization and expression of the stratification-related cytokeratins 4 and 15. *J. Cell Biol.* **106**: 1249.

Mansbridge, J., A.M. Knapp, and A.M. Strefling. 1984. Evidence for an alternative pathway of keratinocyte maturation in psoriasis from an antigen found in psoriatic but not normal epidermis. *J. Invest. Dermatol.* **83**: 296.

Nelson, W.G. and T.-T. Sun. 1983. The 50- and 58-Kdalton keratin classes as molecular markers for stratified squamous epithelia: Cell culture studies. *J. Cell Biol.* **97**: 244.

Rentrop, M., B. Knapp, H. Winter, and J. Schweizer. 1986. Differential localization of distinct keratin mRNA-species in mouse tongue epithelium by in situ hybridization with specific cDNA probes. *J. Cell Biol.* **103**: 2583.

Schermer, A., S. Galvin, and T.-T. Sun. 1986. Differentiation-related expression of a major 64K corneal keratin in vivo and in culture suggests limbal location of corneal epithelial stem cells. *J. Cell Biol.* **103**: 49.

Schweizer, J., M. Kinjo, G. Furstenberger, and H. Winter. 1984. Sequential expression of mRNA encoded keratin sets in neonatal mouse epidermis. *Cell* **37**: 159.

Skerrow, D. and C.J. Skerrow. 1983. Tonofilament differentiation in human epidermis: Isolation and polypeptide chain composition of keratinocyte subpopulations. *Exp. Cell Res.* **143**: 27.

Stoler, A., R. Kopan, M. Duvic, and E. Fuchs. 1988. Use of monospecific antisera and cRNA probes to localize the major changes in keratin expression during normal and abnormal epidermal differentiation. *J. Cell Biol.* **107**: 427.

Sun, T.-T. and H. Green. 1977. Cultured epithelial cells of cornea, conjunctiva and skin: Absence of marked intrinsic divergence of their differentiated states. *Nature* **269**: 489.

Sun, T.-T., R. Eichner, A. Schermer, D. Cooper, W.G. Nelson, and R.A. Weiss. 1984. Classification, expression, and possible mechanisms of evolution of mammalian epithelial keratins: A unifying model. *Cancer Cells* **1**: 167.

Tseng, S.C.G., D. Hatchell, N. Tierney, S.J.W. Huang, and T.-T. Sun. 1984. Expression of specific keratin markers by rabbit corneal, conjunctival and esophageal epithelia during vitamin A deficiency. *J. Cell Biol.* **99**: 2279.

Weiss, R.A., R. Eichner, and T.-T. Sun. 1984. Monoclonal antibody analysis of keratin expression in epidermal diseases: A 48 kd and a 56 kd keratin as molecular markers for hyperproliferative keratinocytes. *J. Cell Biol.* **98**: 1397.

Woodcock-Mitchell, J., R. Eichner, W.G. Nelson, and T.-T. Sun. 1982. Immunolocalization of keratin polypeptides in human epidermis using monoclonal antibodies. *J. Cell Biol.* **95**: 580.

Keratin Proteins:
Diagnostic Aids in Neoplasia

S.P. Banks-Schlegel

Division of Lung Diseases, National Heart, Lung, and Blood Institute
National Institutes of Health, Bethesda, Maryland 20892

All cells contain intermediate filaments (IFs) as part of their cytoskeleton, and the type of IF expressed is characteristic of the cell type (for review, see Moll et al. 1982). Keratin proteins comprise the IFs found in epithelial cells. There are at least 19 distinct keratin proteins (40–70 kD), and specific subsets can be found in different epithelia. The complexity of keratins has been shown to vary, depending on the type of epithelia, the stage of development and/or differentiation of the cells, and the extrinsic environment of the cells. There is a maintenance of the usual cell-type-specific pattern of IF expression during malignant growth and metastasis, with keratin filaments being retained when epithelial cells are transformed (i.e., carcinomas). We have examined for alterations in the expression of this major differentiation product in neoplasia. Our main efforts have been focused on human epithelia derived from major cancer sites of the body such as esophagus, lung, and skin. Because of advances in the ability to grow human epithelial cells, we also used cell culture to analyze events involved in the process of neoplasia.

Cancer of the human esophagus represents a major cause of death in certain populations throughout the world. We have developed cell lines from human esophageal tumor specimens to facilitate examination of the biologic behavior of this tumor type in vitro. Human esophageal carcinoma cells were found to differ from their normal counterpart in terms of their morphologic appearance, growth properties, and the expression of their keratin proteins (Banks-Schlegel and Quintero 1986a). Using one-dimensional gel analysis in conjunction with polyclonal anti-keratin serum, we observed that, similar to primary esophageal carcinomas, esophageal carcinoma cell lines HCE-1 and HCE-3 showed a dramatic reduction or complete loss of the major 52-kD keratin normally present in human esophageal epithelium and cultured esophageal keratinocytes (Fig. 1).

127

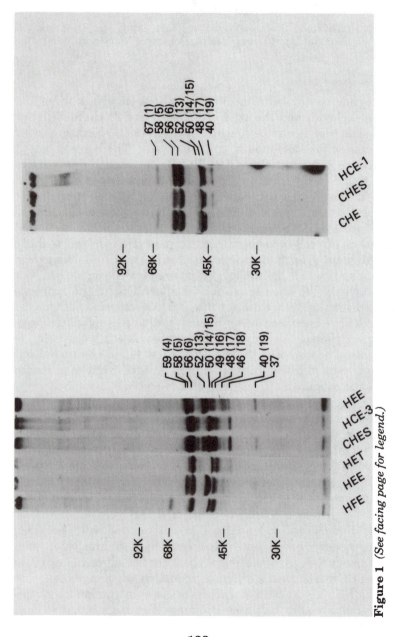

Figure 1 (See facing page for legend.)

128

However, some cell lines exhibited significant levels of the 52-kD keratin (HCE-4, HCE-5, HCE-6, and HCE-7 [NM] derived from an athymic nude mouse tumor initiated from the same primary esophageal carcinoma as the HCE-4 cell line), although it was usually reduced in amounts compared with normal human esophageal cells; one cell line, HCE-1, was observed to synthesize a 67-kD keratin, characteristic of cornifying stratified squamous epithelium such as epidermis. HCE-8 was unique in that it synthesized mainly small-sized keratins (40–50 kD). Hence, although keratin expression is maintained in these epithelial cells following neoplastic transformation, the program of keratin expression is altered. Keratin expression in the cell lines revealed a greater variability in the spectrum of keratins associated with neoplasia than had been observed in primary carcinomas. The lack of expression of certain keratins could be a reflection of the state of differentiation of the cells, cell selection, cell type heterogeneity, and/or other factors.

Growth of human keratinocytes is dependent on epidermal growth factor (EGF). Because EGF receptor number has been shown to be elevated in all squamous cell carcinoma (SQC) cells examined so far, thus suggesting its role in growth control, we analyzed normal and transformed human esophageal epithelial cells for differential sensitivity to EGF. Transformed esophageal cells, although being maximally stimulated by concentrations of EGF similar to normal cells, were not inhibited by higher concentrations of EGF (data not shown) (Banks-Schlegel and Quintero 1986b). This biologic response contrasts with that of other SQC cell lines (e.g., A431 and SCC-15), in which the addition of any EGF to the medium beyond that normally present in serum inhibited cell growth markedly. Because of these differences in the biologic response of the normal

Figure 1 Keratin expression by human esophageal carcinoma cell lines HCE-1 and HCE-3. Radiolabeled keratins were selectively immunoprecipitated from normal and tumor cell extracts with keratin antiserum and analyzed on an 8.5% polyacrylamide gel. (*Left*) Molecular weight markers; (*right*) molecular weights ascribed to the keratins of human esophageal epithelium (HEE) and HCE-1. Numbers in parentheses indicate the probable identity of the keratins according to the nomenclature of Moll et al. (1982). (HFE) Human foreskin epidermis; (HET) a moderately differentiated human esophageal tumor; (CHE and CHES) cultured human epidermal and esophageal keratinocytes, respectively. Data from Banks-Schlegel and Quintero (1986a).

Table 1 Estimated Affinity and Number of EGF Receptors on Human Esophageal Carcinoma Cell Lines

Cell or cell line	kD (nM)	Receptors x10³/cell
Esophageal keratinocytes	16.8	400
Esophageal carcinoma cell lines		
HCE-8	1.1	170
HCU-18	0.9	100
TE-3	0.4	92
HCU-39	1.2	89
TE-2	1.1	87
TE-1	1.0	74
HCU-13	0.6	62
TE-4	1.7	60
HCE-7(NM)	0.6	52
HCE-9	2.7	49
HCE-4	0.5	48
HCE-5	0.8	39
HCE-6	0.3	19
HCE-3	0.2	4

Determined by Scatchard analysis. The experimental values were fit to a single line using linear regression, and all lines had correlation coefficients >0.92. Each Scatchard plot represents the analysis of ten different EGF concentrations (in duplicate). Data from Banks-Schlegel and Quintero (1986b).

and transformed cells to EGF, we looked at receptor level and affinity of the receptors in normal and transformed esophageal epithelial cells. In contrast to results reported for other SQCs, esophageal carcinoma cells were found to have fewer receptors with increased affinity, indicating that squamous cell neoplasia is not dependent on elevated numbers of EGF receptors and that EGF receptor number may have a determinant role in EGF cell toxicity (Table 1). These properties may serve as useful diagnostic markers for human esophageal carcinoma cells.

To determine whether there are specific chromosomal changes associated with human esophageal cancer, we undertook karyotypic analyses of human esophageal carcinoma cell lines. Structural abnormalities in chromosomes 1, 3, and/or 11 were found to be present in all 14 cell lines examined (data not shown). Because the location of the defect on chromosome 11 was the same for most of the cell lines (11 out of 14) (involving the deletion of the p-arm of chromosome 11), the association of chromosome 11 with human esophageal cancer is thought to be of greatest importance (J. Whang-Peng and S. Banks-Schlegel, unpubl.).

Table 2 Distribution of Keratin Proteins in Human Lung Cancer Cell Lines

Cell type	Distribution of keratin proteins with the following molecular weights[a]								
	40,000 (19)[b]	46,000 (18)	48,000 (17)	49,000 (16)	50,000 (14/15)	52,000 (8/13)	54,000 (7)	56,000 (6)	58,000 (5)
SqC (3)[c]	++	(+)	++	(+)	++	(+)	(+)	+++[d]	+++[d]
Mucoepidermoid (1)	+	+	+++	(+)	++	+	+	+++	+++
AC (7)	++	(+)	++	(+)	+	++	+	–[e]	–[e]
LCC (2)	++	(+)	++	(+)	+	++	+	–	–
SCLC (12)	(+)	(+)	+	(+)	+	++	–	–[f]	–[g]
Mesothelioma (4)	++	(+)	+++	(+)	+	+++	+	–	–[h]

Data from Banks-Schlegel et al. (1985).

[a]Graded – to +++ on the basis of intensity on immunoprecipitation; (+) variably present in small amounts.

[b]Numbers in parentheses indicate probable identity of the keratins according to the nomenclature of Moll et al. (1982).

[c]Numbers in parentheses, number examined.

[d]Amount varied, depending on the extent of squamous differentiation with more differentiated cell lines containing more keratin.

[e]One of seven AC cell lines exhibited small amounts of an M_r 58,000 keratin and minute amounts of an M_r 56,000 keratin.

[f]One of 12 SCLC cell lines, NCI-H378, contained a prominent M_r 56,000 keratin at early passage, which was lost upon subsequent passaging. Xenotransplants of this line (from earlier passaged cells) had a mixed SCLC-squamous cell histology.

[g]One of 12 SCLC cell lines, NCI-H60, possessed a prominent M_r 58,000 keratin.

[h]Two of four mesothelioma cell lines contained a prominent M_r 58,000 keratin.

131

Human lung tumors can be divided into four major types: SQC, adenocarcinoma (AC), large cell carcinoma (LCC), and small cell lung carcinoma (SCLC). Using selective immunoprecipitation of labeled extracts with antiserum to total keratin and one-dimensional gel analysis, we examined human lung tumor cell lines established from the major histological types of lung cancer, as well as mesotheliomas, for their pattern of keratin expression (Table 2) (Banks-Schlegel et al. 1985). Small-sized keratins (40–52 kD) were observed in cell lines derived from both SCLC and non-SCLC types of lung cancer. Tumor cell lines exhibiting squamous differentiation by light microscope criteria (i.e., intracellular keratin, intercellular bridging, "pearl" formation, and/or individual cell keratinization) also displayed a preponderance of intermediate-sized keratins (56 and 58 kD), consistent with findings using tumor tissue. Mesothelioma cell lines had varying keratin profiles; some mesothelioma cell lines possessed intermediate-sized keratins (58 kD), as well as small-sized keratins (40–52 kD). The inability to detect high-molecular-mass keratins (>60 kD) in mesothelioma cell lines, in contrast to the strong reactivity of the native tumor with anti-63-kD keratin serum (Said et al. 1983), may be attributed to the fact that high-molecular-mass keratins are frequently suppressed in tissue culture. In this regard, examination of keratin proteins in four cases of mesothelioma by one-dimensional gel electrophoresis following selective immunoprecipitation of labeled extracts with antiserum to total keratins revealed the presence of intermediate-sized keratins and/or high-molecular-mass keratins (>60 kD) in several of the tumors (Fig. 2). All mesotheliomas exhibited keratins in the 40–52-kD range. These studies indicated that demonstration of the presence of intermediate-sized keratins (56 and 58 kD) and/or high-molecular-mass keratins (>60 kD) in mesothelioma cells may be helpful in differentiating mesotheliomas from ACs that are negative for these particular keratins. The presence of keratins in all SCLC cell lines examined argues against a neuroectodermal origin for these tumors and is consistent with the notion that these tumors arise from a common bronchial "stem cell," similar to that from which other types of bronchogenic carcinomas arise.

In human epidermis, distinct keratin domains have been shown with antiserum to small-sized keratins (45 and 46 kD) being localized to the basal layer, whereas staining with antiserum to larger keratins (55 and 63 kD) correlated with the

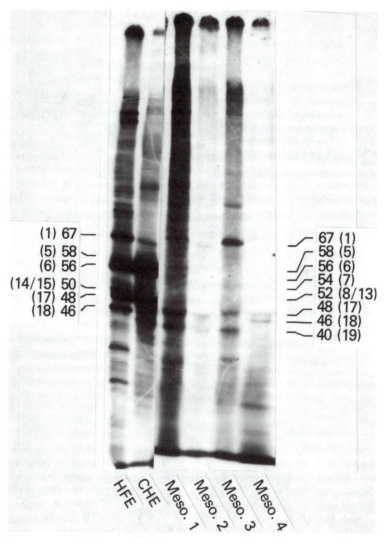

Figure 2 Analysis of keratin proteins from human malignant mesotheliomas. Radiolabeled keratins from human foreskin epidermis (HFE) and cultured human epidermal (CHE) keratinocytes (included as controls), and four cases of malignant mesothelioma (designated Meso. 1, Meso. 2, Meso. 3, and Meso. 4) were selectively immunoprecipitated with antiserum to total keratins purified from human stratum corneum and analyzed on an 8.5% SDS-polyacrylamide gel. Molecular weights (x10⁻³) ascribed to keratins of HFE and the mesothelioma cells are shown to the *left* and *right* of the gel, respectively. Numbers in parenthesis indicate the probable identity of the keratins according to the nomenclature of Moll et al. (1982).

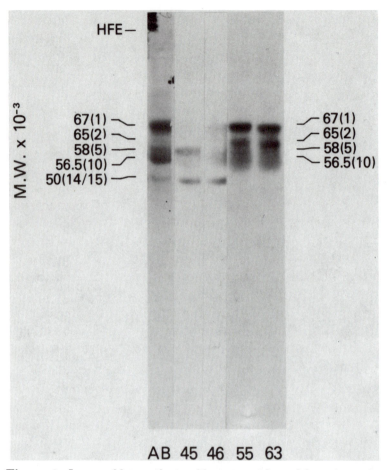

Figure 3 Immunoblot analysis of human epidermal keratins using antibodies to the 45-, 46-, 55-, and 63-kD keratins purified from human callus. Keratins, extracted from human foreskin epidermis (HFE), were resolved on an 8.5% polyacrylamide gel and analyzed by immunoblotting using the anti-45-, ant-46-, anti-55-, and anti-63-kD keratin antibodies. (*Left*) Molecular weights (x10^{-3}) assigned to the epidermal keratins detected on amido black (AB) staining of the nitrocellulose strip; (*right*) those detected following reactivity with antiserum to the 63-kD human callus keratin. Numbers in parentheses represent the probable identity of the keratins according to the nomenclature used by Moll et al. (1982). (45, 46, 55, 63) Molecular weights (x10^{-3}) of the various human callus keratins used as immunogens.

commitment to terminal differentiation and localized predominantly in the suprabasal layers (Banks-Schlegel et al. 1981). Immunoblot analysis of keratins from human foreskin epidermis, performed using serum against the 45-, 46-, 55-, and 63-kD keratins of human callus, demonstrated that the anti-45-kD keratin serum recognized predominantly the 50- and 58-kD keratins, whereas the anti-46-kD keratin serum detected primarily the 50-kD keratin (Fig. 3). The localization of these keratins to the basal layer has also been reported by others (Nelson and Sun 1983). The anti-55- and anti-63-kD keratin sera detected largely the high-molecular-mass keratins (>60 kD), characteristic mainly of keratinizing stratified squamous epithelia. Despite similar patterns of reactivity by Western blot, the pattern of immunocytochemical staining of a variety of squamous tumors using these two antibodies was found to be different, with the anti-55-kD keratin serum staining areas of squamous differentiation and the anti-63-kD keratin serum staining areas of keratinization. Profiles of immunocytochemical staining, using keratin antiserum against these individual keratins (45, 46, 55, and 63 kD), were evaluated in basal cell and SQCs of the human skin and surrounding epidermis (Fig. 4). The specific staining pattern was maintained in SQCs of the skin and other body sites (data not shown; see Thomas et al. 1984). Invasive SQCs, stained with antisera to small-sized keratins (45 and 46 kD), exhibited diffuse staining for the 55-kD keratin and showed focal staining, with antisera to the large keratin (63 kD) being restricted to differentiated areas of tumors in the center of the tumor mass. As expected, basal cell carcinomas stained for small-sized keratins, with no apparent staining for larger keratins (55 and 63 kD) except for focal staining localized to areas of keratinization. These findings suggest that staining for different molecular mass keratins may be helpful in the differential diagnosis of skin lesions. Abnormal keratin profiles were also observed in histologically normal-appearing or hyperplastic epidermis adjacent to SQCs and overlying basal cell carcinomas. Epidermis adjacent to SQCs and basal cell carcinomas showed diffuse staining of all cell layers with antiserum to low-molecular-mass keratins (45 and 46 kD) (usually a predominantly basal staining pattern) and a decreased intensity of suprabasal staining for high-molecular-mass keratin (63 kD). This altered pattern of keratin staining could be due to abnormal squamous maturation, increased rate of cell turnover, response of the adjacent epidermis to the tumor microenvironment, or other factors.

In summary, immunocytochemistry and immunoprecipitation studies utilizing keratin markers in the analysis of normal

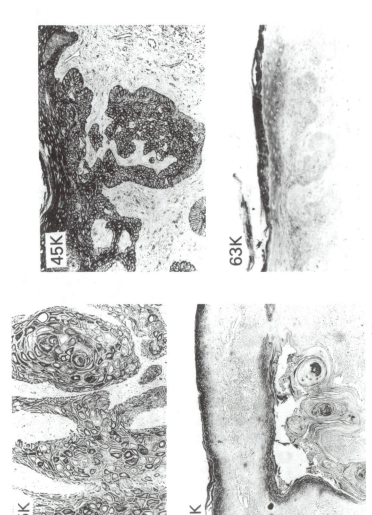

Figure 1 *(See facing page for legend.)*

136

and neoplastic tissues indicated their usefulness in the diagnosis and classification of tumors and in histogenesis.

ACKNOWLEDGMENT

We are grateful to Dorothy Viener for typing the manuscript.

REFERENCES

Banks-Schlegel, S.P. and J. Quintero. 1986a. Growth and differentiation of human esophageal carcinoma cell lines. *Cancer Res.* **46:** 250.
————. 1986b. Human esophageal carcinoma cells have fewer, but higher affinity epidermal growth factor receptors. *J. Biol. Chem.* **261:** 4359.
Banks-Schlegel, S.P., A.F. Gazdar, and C.C. Harris. 1985. Intermediate filament and cross-linked envelope expression in human lung tumor cell lines. *Cancer Res.* **45:** 1187.
Banks-Schlegel, S.P., R. Schlegel, and G.S. Pinkus. 1981. Keratin protein domains within the human epidermis. *Exp. Cell Res.* **136:** 465.
Moll, R., W.W. Franke, D.L. Schiller, B. Geiger, and R. Krepler. 1982. The catalog of human cytokeratins: Patterns of expression in normal epithelia, tumors and cultured cells. *Cell* **31:** 11.
Nelson, W.G. and T.-T. Sun. 1983. The 50- and 58-kdalton keratin classes as molecular markers for stratified squamous epithelia: Cell culture studies. *J. Cell Biol.* **97:** 244.
Said, J.W., G. Nash, S. Banks-Schlegel, A.F. Sassoon, S. Murakami, and P. Shintaku. 1983. Keratin in human lung tumors. Patterns of localization of different-molecular-weight keratin proteins. *Am. J. Pathol.* **113:** 27.
Thomas, P., J.W. Said, G. Nash, and S. Banks-Schlegel. 1984. Profiles of keratin proteins in basal and squamous cell carcinoma of the skin. *Lab. Invest.* **50:** 36.

Figure 4 Immunoperoxidase staining of an invasive squamous cell carcinoma and a basal cell carcinoma of the skin with antiserum to the 45-kD and 63-kD keratins. (*Left*) Invasive squamous cell carcinoma stained with antiserum to 45-kD (*top*) and 63-kD (*bottom*) keratins. Staining for the 63-kD keratin is localized to the keratinized areas of the tumor (black). (*Right*) Basal cell carcinoma stained with antiserum to 45-kD (*top*) and 63-kD (*bottom*) keratins. Whereas diffuse staining for the 45-kD keratin was observed, no staining of the basal cell carcinoma for the 63-kD keratin was noted despite staining of the more highly differentiated cells in the overlying epidermis (black). Methyl green counterstain.

Cytoskeletal Markers in the Classification of Carcinomas and Their Metastases

R. Moll

Institute of Pathology, University of Mainz
Mainz, Federal Republic of Germany

Although intermediate filaments are morphologically inconspicuous cytoplasmic structures, their study has resulted in a major advance in diagnostic tumor pathology on the basis of the cell-type-specific expression of the various intermediate filament subunits. Of these structures, the cytokeratins (CKs), i.e., the epithelial type of intermediate filaments, are worthy of particular attention because of their high degree of diversity. In the various human epithelia (excluding "hard" keratins of hair- and nail-forming cells), 19 distinct CK polypeptides have been identified so far (Franke et al. 1981; Moll et al. 1982; Tseng et al. 1982), and these are expressed in different cell-type-specific combinations. By analyzing these proteins biochemically, using two-dimensional gel electrophoresis, we have found different CK patterns in different carcinoma types (Moll et al. 1982; Moll and Franke 1986). In many cases, these patterns are typical for specific kinds of carcinomas and are also maintained in their metastases. For example, squamous cell carcinomas of different origin are characterized by the predominance of a particular set of CKs typical of stratified epithelia, notably, CKs 5, 6, and 14–17. This distinctive feature allows their positive identification as squamous cell tumors, even when the degree of differentiation is very low (Moll et al. 1982; Nelson et al. 1984; Moll and Franke 1986).

In the following text, some recent findings concerning CK typing in transitional cell carcinomas and adenocarcinomas are presented.

Transitional Cell Carcinomas

Among the various epithelial tissues, the urothelium is unique with respect not only to its morphological features, but also to its CK expression pattern. Although the set of the four simple epithelium-type CKs (7, 8, 18, and 19) is expressed throughout all urothelial cell layers, the stratification-related components CKs 5 and 17 appear to be restricted to the basal cell layer, and, even more striking, CK 13 is abundantly expressed in the basal and intermediate cells but ceases to be detectable in the superficial polar "umbrella" cells (Moll et al. 1988).

This complex CK expression pattern points to a bimodality of differentiation and probably reflects the intrinsic capacity of this epithelium to change its character, toward either glandular or squamous metaplasia.

In a recent study of urothelium-derived carcinomas, we found several types of CK patterns (Moll et al. 1988). Although transitional cell carcinomas (TCCs) of grade 1 resemble the normal urothelium rather closely, grade-2 carcinomas exhibit some deviations. TCCs of grade 3, including metastases, prominently and mainly express the four simple epithelial CKs 7, 8, 18, and 19. Although poor differentiation is accompanied by very low levels of CK 13 in G3 tumors, immunohistochemistry does reveal the presence of some scattered individual cells expressing CK 13 in most such tumors and their metastases. Squamous metaplasia results in an increase in stratification-related CKs; nevertheless, urothelial features such as CKs 7 and 13 are usually still maintained. The CK profile of TCCs, which is characterized by prominent amounts of CKs 7, 8, 18, and 19, together with varying amounts of CK 13 as well as "IT protein" (see below), may help to confirm a urothelial origin in diagnostically unclear carcinoma cases (poor differentiation, metastases).

Adenocarcinomas
Carcinomas of the simple epithelial type, including the various adenocarcinomas, comprise a large spectrum of different tumors, and the majority of diagnostic problem cases fall into this category. Among these tumors, the diversity of CK patterns is rather limited, with only three major patterns being distinguishable (CKs 8, 18; CKs 8, 18, 19; CKs 7, 8, 18, 19). Some diagnostic information can be obtained by testing for CK 7 (see Moll et al. 1982; Moll and Franke 1986; Osborn et al. 1986; see also van Eyken et al. 1988).

We have been searching for other cytoskeletal proteins that might enable certain adenocarcinomas to be distinguished from one another. In two-dimensional gel electrophoretic analyses, we have observed a particular cytoskeletal protein with an apparent molecular weight of 46,000 and an isoelectric point of pH 6.1 (designated IT protein; Moll et al. 1982), which appears to be present in intestinal epithelium, in corresponding adenocarcinomas of colon, in the HT-29 colon carcinoma cell line, and, surprisingly, in Merkel cell tumors of the skin (Moll and Franke 1985). Although IT protein was found to react with an antiserum against a bovine epidermal prekeratin (Moll and Franke 1985), its relationship to the CKs remained open to question, particularly as negative reactions were obtained with a large series of other established CK antibodies, as well as with the anti-intermediate filament antibody of Pruss et al. (1981).

In contrast, however, we have recently observed that IT protein reacts positively with the general CK antibody lu-5 (R. Moll and W.W. Franke, in prep.). In a nitrocellulose blot-binding assay (Hatzfeld et al. 1987), radiolabeled CK 8 bound significantly to IT protein, which thus appears to behave like a type-I CK. In 4 M urea, purified IT protein is also able to form complexes with the type-II CK 8, and intermediate filaments are reconstituted in vitro upon removal of the urea (R. Moll and W.W. Franke, in prep.).

We have raised guinea pig antibodies against IT protein electrophoretically purified from intestinal mucosa. At immunoelectron microscopy, this antibody was observed to bind to CK filaments of HT-29 cells. Immunocytochemical screening of a large series of normal human tissues revealed a strong positive reaction in intestinal epithelial cells (Fig. 1a,b), as well as in the foveolar epithelium of the stomach mucosa, the superficial (umbrella) cells of the transitional epithelium, and the Merkel cells of the epidermis. Mosaic-like patterns indicating heterogeneity of intercellular staining were often conspicuous. Some other epithelia such as that of the gall bladder contained a few positive cells. Most of the other epithelia studied, including a variety of simple epithelia, were negative (R. Moll and W.W. Franke, in prep.).

The distribution of IT protein in human carcinomas reflects the normal pattern rather closely. Thus, all of the 23 cases of adenocarcinoma of the colon studied were positive for IT protein, the staining pattern being either uniform or heterogeneous (Fig. 2). Expression of IT protein was also found in the majority of adenocarcinomas of the stomach, pancreas, and gall bladder, in most transitional cell carcinomas, as well as in all

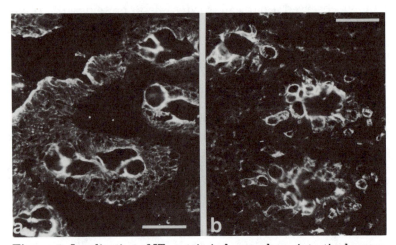

Figure 1 Localization of IT protein in human large intestinal mucosa ([a] surface zone; [b] crypt zone; frozen sections), using indirect immunofluorescence microscopy (guinea pig antibodies specific for IT protein). Note the uniformly positive reaction of the surface epithelium (enterocytes and goblet cells) and of the necks of the crypts (a) but a heterogeneous mosaic-like staining pattern of the deeper crypt epithelium (b). Bars, 50 μm.

Merkel cell carcinomas studied; in contrast, most carcinomas from other sites, including adenocarcinomas, were completely negative (R. Moll and W.W. Franke, in prep.).

These results show that the expression spectrum of IT protein is much more restricted than are the spectra of the established simple epithelial CKs. Thus, IT protein would seem to be a very promising diagnostic marker for the differential diagnosis of various simple epithelial tumors; e.g., IT protein should be valuable in distinguishing adenocarcinomas of the gastrointestinal tract from adenocarcinomas of the breast, lung, or endometrium, as the latter are negative for IT protein.

The question remains whether IT protein is a new CK protein. The data presented here show that IT protein fulfills many of the criteria used to classify a type-I CK of the simple epithelial group; most important, IT protein is able to reconstitute intermediate filaments in combination with a type-II CK in vitro. Therefore, it seems appropriate to add this protein to CKs 18 and 19 and tentatively designate it as CK 20. The definitive classification, however, must await the availability of amino acid sequence data.

In conclusion, CK typing of epithelial tumors already has an

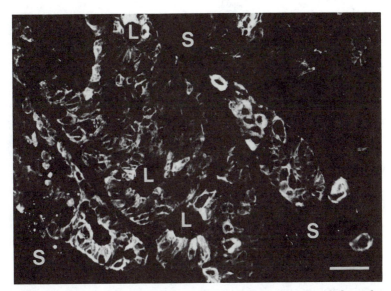

Figure 2   Ovarian metastasis of an adenocarcinoma of the colon strongly positive for IT protein (frozen section; indirect immunofluorescence microscopy using guinea pig antibodies).   Note the heterogeneous staining pattern. (L) Lumina of tubular tumor structures; (S) stroma. Bar, 50 μm.

important place in carcinoma diagnosis, often allowing a more precise classification of metastatic tumor diseases. Still lacking is a sufficient number of selective CK antibodies that can be successfully applied to paraffin sections. Up to now, only CKs 8, 13, and 19 can be detected in routinely prepared material. Hopefully, in the future more such reagents will be developed that would enable a broader application of CK typing under routine conditions.

ACKNOWLEDGMENTS

The technical assistance of Christine Zech, Jutta Jacobi, and Ulrike Hesse is gratefully acknowledged. Thanks are also due to Helga Breitbach and Karin Molter for photographic work and to Christine Bürkner for typing of the manuscript.

REFERENCES
Franke, W.W., D.L. Schiller, R. Moll, S. Winter, S. Schmid, I. Engelbrecht, H. Denk, R. Krepler, and B. Platzer. 1981. Diversity of

cytokeratins. Differentiation specific expression of cytokeratin polypeptides in epithelial cells and tissues. *J. Mol. Biol.* **153**: 933.

Hatzfeld, M., G. Maier, and W.W. Franke. 1987. Cytokeratin domains involved in heterotopic complex formation determined by in-vitro binding assays. *J. Mol. Biol.* **197**: 237.

Moll, R. and W.W. Franke. 1985. Cytoskeletal differences between human neuroendocrine tumors. A cytoskeletal protein of molecular weight 46,000 distinguishes cutaneous from pulmonary neuroendocrine neoplasms. *Differentiation* **30**: 165.

―――. 1986. Cytochemical cell typing of metastatic tumors according to their cytoskeletal proteins. In *Biochemistry and molecular genetics of cancer metastasis* (ed. K. Lapis et al.), p. 101. Nijhoff, The Hague.

Moll, R., W.W. Franke, D.L. Schiller, B. Geiger, and R. Krepler. 1982. The catalog of human cytokeratins: Patterns of expression in normal epithelia, tumors and cultured cells. *Cell* **31**: 11.

Moll, R., T. Achtstätter, E. Becht, J. Balcarova-Ständer, M. Ittensohn, and W.W. Franke. 1988. Cytokeratins in normal and malignant transitional epithelium: Maintenance of expression of urothelial differentiation features in transitional cell carcinomas and bladder carcinoma cell lines. *Am. J. Pathol.* **132**: 123.

Nelson, W.G., H. Battifora, H. Santana, and T.-T. Sun. 1984. Specific cytokeratins as molecular markers for neoplasms with a stratified epithelial origin. *Cancer Res.* **44**: 1600.

Osborn, M., G. Van Lessen, K. Weber, G. Klöppel, and M. Altmannsberger. 1986. Differential diagnosis of gastrointestinal carcinomas by using monoclonal antibodies specific for individual keratin polypeptides. *Lab. Invest.* **55**: 497.

Pruss, R.M., R. Mirsky, M.C. Ruff, R. Thorpe, A.J. Dowding, and B.H. Anderton. 1981. All classes of intermediate filaments share a common antigenetic determinant defined by a monoclonal antibody. *Cell* **27**: 419.

Tseng, S.C.G., M.J. Jarvinen, W.G. Nelson, J.-W. Huang, J. Woodcock-Mitchell, and T.-T. Sun. 1982. Correlation of specific keratins with different types of epithelial differentiation: Monoclonal antibody studies. *Cell* **30**: 361.

Van Eyken, P., R. Sciot, A. Paterson, F. Callea, M.C. Kew, and V.J. Desmet. 1988. Cytokeratin expression in hepatocellular carcinoma: An immunohistochemical study. *Hum. Pathol.* **19**: 562.

Keratin Patterns
in Epithelial Tumors

H.J. Kahn and R. Baumal

Departments of Pathology, Women's College Hospital
The Hospital for Sick Children
The University of Toronto, Toronto, Ontario, Canada

Keratins are 10-nm intermediate filaments that have proved to be very useful in the diagnosis of tumors. They are expressed in all normal epithelia and in neoplasms derived from these epithelia, including tumors both well and poorly differentiated (Osborn and Weber 1983; Kahn et al. 1984). Patterns of keratin distribution play an important role (1) in differentiating epithelial from nonepithelial tumors such as lymphomas, malignant melanomas, and sarcomas; (2) in differentiating one type of epithelial neoplasm from another (Huszar et al. 1986); and (3) in the case of metastatic adenocarcinomas of unknown origin, suggesting the primary site. The different patterns of keratin distribution that could be of diagnostic siginificance in addressing the above questions would be (1) the type of keratin expression in the tumor, on the basis of molecular weight and isoelectric point (Moll et al. 1982); (2) the pattern of arrangement of keratin filaments in the cell (Corson and Pinkus 1982; Kahn et al. 1982, 1986); and (3) the coexpression of keratin with other filaments (Yeger et al. 1986; Azumi and Battifora 1987).

We performed immunoperoxidase staining using a number of different keratin antibodies on formalin-fixed histological material and cytological preparations from effusions and needle aspirates on a large number of primary and metastatic tumors to see whether patterns of keratin distribution could differentiate epithelial from nonepithelial tumors and differentiate different types of epithelial tumors and to assess whether the primary site of a metastatic adenocarcinoma could be ascertained.

Type of Keratin Expression in the Tumor
Of the 19 subtypes of keratins that have been identified, antibodies are available that recognize high-molecular-weight keratins, seen in squamous epithelium and squamous cell carcinomas, as well as low-molecular weight keratins, which can

145

Table 1 Distribution of Filaments in Different Epithelial Tumors

Type of tumor	Antibody[a]				
	HMK	LMK	Vi	NF	actin
Squamous cell carcinoma	+	–	–	–	–
Mesothelioma	+	+	+	–	–
Adenocarcinomas					
breast	+	+	–	–	+ (diffuse)
colon	–	+	–	–	+ (apical)
lung	±	+	±	–	+ (diffuse)
kidney	–	+	+	–	–
thyroid	+	+	+	–	–
ovarian/ endometrial	–	+	+	–	–
stomach	–	+	–	–	± (apical)
Neuroendocrine					
carcinoid	–	+	–	–	–
Merkel	–	+	–	+	–
oat cell	–	+	–	±	–
Synovial sarcoma	–	+	+	–	–
Thymoma	+	–	–	–	–
Pleomorphic adenoma	+	+	+	–	–

[a](HMK) High-molecular-weight keratin; (LMK) low-molecular-weight keratin; (Vi) vimentin; (NF) neurofilament; (+) positive; (–) negative; (±) some cases positive.

be detected in virtually all simple epithelia, most adenocarcinomas, and transitional cell carcinomas (Table 1) (Moll et al. 1982, 1988; Chan et al. 1988). Our results confirmed that the high-molecular-weight keratins were detected mainly in well-differentiated and poorly differentiated squamous cell carcinomas, and also in a few adenocarcinomas, such as breast and papillary thyroid carcinomas, and occasionally at the invasive edge of other types of adenocarcinomas. Some mesotheliomas also expressed high-molecular-weight keratins. Low-molecular-weight keratins were detected in adenocarcinomas, mesotheliomas, and neuroendocrine tumors. Specific subtypes of keratin have been noted in some tumors such as cytokeratin 5 in mesotheliomas (Blobel et al. 1985) and cytokeratin 7 in cholangiocellular carcinomas (Fisher et al. 1987).

Table 2 Distribution of Keratin Filaments within the Cell

Pattern	Diagnosis
Perinuclear	mesothelioma
Peripheral or web	adenocarcinoma
Punctate dot or crescent	neuroendocrine (carcinoid Merkel)
Diffuse	adenocarcinoma, mesothelioma, neuroendocrine

Patterns of Arrangement of Keratin Filaments within a Tumor Cell

Several different patterns of keratin distribution within a tumor cell were of diagnostic significance (Table 2). A perinuclear pattern of keratin distribution, often associated with juxtanuclear condensation of keratin filaments, was seen in the epithelial type of mesothelioma in both cytological specimens and tissue sections. This pattern of arrangement was also seen in preparations containing normal and reactive mesothelial cells. Tumor cells required abundant cytoplasm for this pattern to be appreciated by the immunoperoxidase techniques. However, this pattern could still be discerned ultrastructurally in the more spindle-shaped mesothelial cells. In addition, in cases where the pattern is discernible by light microscopy, it could be obscured by prolongation of staining in the chromogen.

In adenocarcinomas arising at different sites, several patterns of keratin filament distribution could be detected. A peripheral pattern along the plasma membrane could be detected in some adenocarcinomas, especially colonic and ovarian adenocarcinomas. In some cases, there was apical accentuation of the filaments, particularly along the luminal border of tumor cells forming glands. In a number of adenocarcinomas, a web-like pattern of keratin filaments could be seen, similar to that detected by immunofluorescence of keratin filaments. If the immunoperoxidase reaction was allowed to continue for too long, the pattern was obscured with the formation of diffuse cytoplasmic staining.

In some carcinoid tumors, all Merkel cell tumors, and some cases of oat cell carcinoma, keratin filaments were arranged in the form of punctate dots or crescents within the cytoplasm. In both carcinoid tumors and oat cell carcinomas, the pattern of distribution of the keratin could be obscured by prolonged incubation with the chromogen. This, however, did not occur with the Merkel cell tumor.

Coexpression of Keratin with Other Filaments

Coexpression of keratin filaments with other types of intermediate filaments, or actin, was useful in differentiating one type of epithelial tumor from another (Table 1). Mesotheliomas and pleomorphic adenomas coexpressed with keratin and vimentin, whereas most adenocarcinomas did not, with the exception of renal, thyroid, ovarian, and small numbers of lung adenocarcinomas. Breast carcinomas often expressed high-molecular-weight keratins and showed diffuse actin staining, whereas the colonic adenocarcinomas expressed low-molecular-weight keratin and showed apical staining with antibody to actin. Gastric adenocarcinomas arising from glands showing colonic metaplasia also showed apical staining with antibody to actin. Metastases of these tumors demonstrated a similar distribution of filaments. In the case of a metastasis from an unknown primary, the distribution of filaments helped to delineate the origin of the tumor. This was particularly useful on formalin-fixed material, since fewer types of adenocarcinomas coexpressed keratin and vimentin than has been demonstrated on alcohol-fixed or frozen material.

Our results confirm that keratin antibodies differentiate epithelial from nonepithelial tumors. Antibodies to high-molecular-weight keratins were demonstrated in squamous cell carcinomas and squamous metaplastic areas, as shown by ourselves and others (Huszar et al. 1986). In contrast, low-molecular-weight keratins were detected in adenocarcinomas, mesotheliomas, and neuroendocrine tumors. Specific cytoplasmic arrangement of keratin filaments could be detected in reactive mesothelial cells and mesotheliomas (Corson and Pinkus 1982; Kahn et al. 1982, 1986; Montag et al. 1988), adenocarcinomas (Kahn et al. 1986; Chan et al. 1988), carcinoid, and Merkel cell tumors (Kahn et al. 1986; Battifora and Silva 1986).

In metastatic adenocarcinomas of unknown origin, the pattern of filament expression helped to define the site of the primary tumor. The coexpression of either high- or low-molecular-weight keratin filaments, or both, with vimentin delineated mesotheliomas and some types of adenocarcinomas and their metastases. The arrangement of luminal actin filaments in colonic adenocarcinomas differentiated these tumors and their metastases from most other types of adenocarcinomas and their metastases.

ACKNOWLEDGMENTS
The authors thank W. Chan and I. Leites for their excellent technical assistance and P. Dickenson for typing the manuscript.

REFERENCES
Azumi, N. and H. Battifora. 1987. The distribution of vimentin and keratin in epithelial and non-epithelial neoplasms. *Am. J. Clin. Pathol.* **88**: 286.

Battifora, H. and E.G. Silva. 1986. The use of antikeratin antibodies in the immunohistochemical distinction between neuroendocrine (Merkel cell) carcinoma of the skin, lymphoma and oat cell carcinoma. *Cancer* **58**: 1040.

Blobel, G.A., R. Moll, W.W. Franke, K.W. Kayser, and V.E. Gould. 1985. The intermediate filament cytoskeleton of malignant mesotheliomas and its diagnostic significance. *Am. J. Pathol.* **121**: 235.

Chan, R., B.F. Edwards, R. Hu, P.V. Rossitto, B.H. Min, J.K. Lund, and R.D. Cardiff. 1988. Characterization of two monoclonal antibodies in an immunohistochemical study of keratin 8 and 18 expression. *Am. J. Clin. Pathol.* **89**: 472.

Corson, J.M. and G.S. Pinkus. 1982. Mesothelioma: Profile of keratin proteins and carcinoembryonic antigen: An immunoperoxidase study of 20 cases and comparison with pulmonary adenocarcinomas. *Am. J. Pathol.* **108**: 80.

Fisher, H.P., M. Altmannsberger, K. Weber, and M. Osborn. 1987. Keratin polypeptides in malignant epithelial liver tumors. Differential diagnostic and histogenetic aspects. *Am. J. Pathol.* **127**: 530.

Huszar, M., O. Gigi-Leitner, R. Moll, W.W. Franke, and B. Geiger. 1986. Monoclonal antibodies to various acidic (type 1) cytokeratins of stratified epithelia. Selective markers for stratification and squamous cell carcinomas. *Differentiation* **31(2)**: 141.

Kahn, H.J., W. Hanna, H. Yeger, and R. Baumal. 1982. Immunohistochemical localization of prekeratin filaments in benign and malignant cells in effusions. *Am. J. Pathol.* **109**: 206.

Kahn, H.J., S.-N. Huang, W. Hanna, R. Baumal, and M.J. Phillips. 1984. Immunohistochemical localization of epidermal and Mallory body cytokeratin in undifferentiated epithelial tumors. *Am. J. Clin. Pathol.* **81**: 184.

Kahn, H.J., P.S. Thorner, H. Yeger, D. Bailey, and R. Baumal. 1986. Distinct keratin patterns demonstrated by immunoperoxidase staining of adenocarcinomas, carcinoids, and mesotheliomas using polyclonal and monoclonal antikeratin antibodies. *Am. J. Clin. Pathol.* **86**: 566.

Moll, R., T. Achtstatter, E. Becht, J. Balcarova-Stander, and W.W. Franke. 1988. Cytokeratins in normal and malignant transitional epithelium. Maintenance of expression of urothelial differentiation features in transitional cell carcinomas and bladder carcinoma cell culture lines. *Am. J. Pathol.* **132(1)**: 123.

Moll, R., W.W. Franke, D.L. Schiller, B. Geiger, and R. Krepler. 1982.

The catalog of human cytokeratins: Patterns of normal epithelia, tumors and cultural cells. *Cell* **31**: 11.

Montag, A.G., G.S. Pinkus, and J.M. Corson. 1988. Keratin protein immunoreactivity of sarcomatoid and mixed types of diffuse malignant mesothelioma. An immunoperoxidase study of 30 cases. *Hum. Pathol.* **19**: 336.

Osborn, M. and K. Weber. 1983. Tumor diagnosis by intermediate filament typing: A novel tool for surgical pathology. *Lab. Invest.* **48**: 372.

Yeger, H., R. Baumal, H.J. Kahn, G. Duwe, and M.J. Phillips. 1986. The use of cytoskeletal characteristics of tumor cells for the diagnosis of colon and breast carcinomas. *Am. J. Clin. Pathol.* **86**: 697.

Cytokeratins and Desmosomal Proteins in Certain Epithelioid and Nonepithelial Cells

W.W. Franke, L. Jahn, and A.C. Knapp

Division of Membrane Biology and Biochemistry, Institute of Cell and
Tumor Biology, German Cancer Research Center
D-6900 Heidelberg, Federal Republic of Germany

Many elements of the vertebrate cytoskeleton, including the
three major kinds of cytoplasmic filaments (microfilaments, microtubules, intermediate-sized filaments [IFs]) and the various
intercellular junctions, occur in structurally similar forms, assembled from different proteins synthesized in cell-type-specific
patterns that are related to certain pathways of differentiation.
Among the different groups of tissues, the epithelia characteristically contain IFs of the cytokeratin category (Franke et al.
1978a,b, 1979e; Sun and Green 1978; Sun et al. 1979; Schlegel
et al. 1980), which are to be distinguished from the other IF
proteins (desmin, vimentin, peripherin, glial filament, and
neurofilament proteins; Franke et al. 1982b; Osborn and Weber
1983; Traub 1985; Steinert and Roop 1987) and junctions of the
desmosome type. The latter are distinguished from the plaque-
bearing adhering junctions of the intermediate type (i.e.,
zonula adhaerens, fascia adhaerens, punctum adhaerens) by
several constitutive polypeptides (Franke et al. 1981b, 1982a,
1987; Cowin and Garrod 1983; Cowin et al. 1985a,b; Steinberg
et al. 1987).

Moreover, the specific sets of cytokeratins and desmosomal
proteins synthesized in different epithelia or in different kinds
of epithelial cells present in the same epithelium can also differ. This diversity is particularly impressive in the case of the
cytokeratins. In human tissues, for example, these represent a
large multigene family of at least 19 epithelial and 10 trichocytic polypeptides (Franke et al. 1981a; Moll et al. 1982; Quinlan et al. 1985; Sun et al. 1985; Heid et al. 1988); similarly,
great complexities have been reported from other vertebrate
species such as cow, rat, mouse, frog, and fish (see, e.g., Franke
et al. 1981a, 1982b; Schiller et al. 1982; Franz et al. 1983;
Cooper and Sun 1986; Markl and Franke 1988). Numerous
studies have shown that a certain cytokeratin polypeptide pattern is typical of a given type of epithelium and that

stoichiometric proportions of cytokeratin polypeptides of the acidic (type I) and basic (type II) subfamilies are required to form typical IFs (for review, see Moll et al. 1982; Quinlan et al. 1985; Sun et al. 1985; Fuchs et al. 1987; Steinert and Roop 1987). Among the various polypeptides identified in desmosomes, some have been established as constitutive desmosome-specific components found in all tissues possessing true desmosomes (i.e., most epithelia, some endothelia and neurothelia, myocardium, reticular cells of thymus and lymph node follicles), notably the cytoplasmic plaque protein, desmoplakin I (Franke et al. 1982a; Mueller and Franke 1983), and the transmembrane glycoprotein, desmoglein (Cowin and Garrod 1983; Giudice et al. 1984; Schmelz et al. 1986a,b). Other desmosomal polypeptides have so far been identified only in certain stratified and complex epithelia (see, e.g., Cowin et al. 1985a; Kapprell et al. 1988).

With the availability of sensitive antibodies specific for desmosomal proteins and individual cytokeratin polypeptides, it has been possible, during recent years, to examine a large number of tissues and cell types of many species, using immunocytochemistry or gel electrophoretic analyses. Most of these studies have confirmed and extended the examples showing the constitutive occurrence of cytokeratin IFs and desmosomes in various kinds of true epithelia, i.e., tissues bordering on both a luminal space and a basal lamina, sometimes in coexistence with IFs containing one or several other IF proteins (for examples, see Franke et al. 1979c,d,f, 1986; Osborn et al. 1980; Achtstätter et al. 1986). In addition, however, several tissues in which cytokeratins and/or desmosomal proteins occur do not display a typical epithelial organization; and some clearly nonepithelial cells, normal as well as malignantly transformed ones, do contain cytokeratins and/or desmosomal proteins. In contrast to the typical epithelial cell types, in which cytokeratin IFs and desmosomes are constitutive and often abundant cell components in all the diverse vertebrate species, many of the epithelioid (epithelium-like) or nonepithelial cells that synthesize cytokeratins show surprising differences of expression between different species and, in some examples, even between different cells of the same tissue.

Epithelioid Tissues
The classification of a given cell or tissue as epithelial is not easy in many instances. In histology textbooks, epithelium is

Table 1 Examples of Epithelioid Tissues without Cytokeratins and/or Desmoplakins

---

Most mammalian and avian endothelia (1)

Chicken retinal pigment "epithelium" (2)

Neurothelia (perineurium and arachnoid) of some higher vertebrates (3)

Ependymal cells of some mammalian species (4)

Mammalian and avian lens "epithelium" (5)

Gonadal and sertoli cells of seminiferous epithelium of mature testis of several mammalian species (6)

Granulosa cells of oocyte follicles of some mammalian species (7)

Adrenal cortex of some species (8)

Epithelioid tissues are formed by one or several layers of laterally connected cells that rest on a basal lamina but are not continuous with the body surface (with the exception of the special case of the composite seminiferous epithelium, which is continuous with the polar epithelia of the rete testis and the ductuli efferentes).

References: (1) Franke et al. (1979b, 1988); Schmid et al. (1979); Fujimoto and Singer (1986). (2) Docherty et al. (1984); Owaribe et al. (1988). (3) Peltonen et al. (1987); Achtstätter et al. (1989). (4) Kasper et al. (1986); Miettinen et al. (1986); see, however, Masters et al. (1985) and Franko et al. (1987). (5) Barritault et al. (1980); Ramaekers et al. (1980); Granger and Lazarides (1984); Alcala and Maisel (1985). (6) Franke et al. (1979a); Van Vorstenbosch et al. (1984); Paranko et al. (1986). (7) Czernobilsky et al. (1985). (8) For example, in rat; for heterogeneous reactions in human adrenal cortex, see Henzen-Logmans et al. (1988).

usually defined as any tissue lining the body surface or a lumen that is continuous with the external space. This definition would include the special case of the testicular germinal epithelium which, in the adult, lacks cytokeratin IFs and desmosomes in many species (see below); it might also be extended to comprise the lining of internal, i.e., coelomic, cavities such as the mesothelium, which, by its structural organization and the constitutive presence of desmosomes and cytokeratin IFs (Franke et al. 1979e; Schmid et al. 1979), often together with vimentin IFs (LaRocca and Rheinwald 1984; Czernobilsky et al. 1985), is a typical epithelium. However, it is difficult to subsume under this definition the cell layer lining the blood and lymph vessels, which is therefore often treated as an epithelioid tissue in its own right, i.e., as endothelium. Interestingly, the vascular endothelium and several other cell-layer-forming tissues that rest on a basal lamina or an equivalent structure (e.g., a fibrous "capsule") but do not border on a free luminal space exhibit remarkable interspecies differences in that they possess cytokeratin IFs and desmosomes in some species but not in others (Table 1).

In lower vertebrates such as amphibia and fish, the entire vascular endothelium appears to be positive for cytokeratins equivalent to human cytokeratins 8 and 18 (see, e.g., Godsave et al. 1986; Jahn et al. 1987; Ferretti et al. 1988; Markl and Franke 1988). In contrast, the endothelium of avian and mammalian species is devoid of cytokeratins and desmosomes, except for two rare subtypes of endothelial cells present in some mammalian tissues, which express some cytokeratin 8 and 18 (Jahn et al. 1987) and desmosomes, respectively (Franke et al. 1988; Table 2), in addition to the predominant vimentin IFs (Franke et al. 1979b).

Differences between species have also been noted in retinal pigment epithelial cells: In amphibia and some mammals, these cells contain desmosomes and cytokeratin IFs, sometimes together with vimentin IFs (Kasper et al. 1988b; McKechnie et al. 1988; Owaribe et al. 1988). In chicken, the same cells are devoid of desmosomes and contain IFs only of the vimentin type (Table 1).

In amphibia, the cells of both neurothelia, i.e., the perineurium of the peripheral nerves and the arachnoid layers of the central nervous system, including the optic nerve, contain desmosomes and IFs of the cytokeratin type (Jahn et al. 1987; Ferretti et al. 1988; Rungger-Brändle et al. 1988; Achtstätter et al. 1989). A similar situation is found in bovine arachnoid cells, which also contain some vimentin IFs (Achtstätter et al. 1989). Bovine and porcine perineurial cells contain cytokeratin IFs

Table 2 Examples of Reticular Tissue Formations of Cells with Certain Epithelial Features in Several Mammalian Species

Reticular epithelium of thymus (various cytokeratins, typical desmosomes) (1)

Dendritic reticulum cells of lymph nodes (desmosomes, no cytokeratins) (2)

Interfollicular reticulum cells of lymph nodes (cytokeratins 8 and 18, no desmosomes) (3)

Sinusoidal reticulum of stellate endothelial cells of lymph nodes (desmosomes, no cytokeratins) (4)

References: (1) Franke et al. (1979e, 1981b, 1982a); Sun et al. (1979); Moll et al. (1983); Laster et al. (1986). (2) Franke and Moll (1987). (3) Franke and Moll (1987). (4) Franke et al. (1988).

(Ortonne et al. 1987; Achtstätter et al. 1989), apparently together with vimentin in some cells, but no desmosomes. In contrast, perineurial cells of human and rat nerves contain only vimentin and no cytokeratin and are also devoid of desmosomes.

The lens epithelium is known to contain only vimentin IFs and no true desmosomes in mammals and birds (Table 1), whereas cytokeratin IFs have been identified in the lens epithelium of a fish, the rainbow trout (Markl and Franke 1988), probably in addition to vimentin IFs.

A developmental change of cytoskeletal complement has been described for the Sertoli cells of rat testes, which contain both cytokeratin IFs and desmosomes in fetal stages but only vimentin IFs and nondesmosomal junctions in the adult (Franke et al. 1979a; Paranko et al. 1986), a situation also found in normal adult testes of some other mammalian species (Table 1).

From all these examples of profound interspecies differences, one is forced to conclude that neither desmosomes nor cytokeratins are essential for the basic functions of these epithelioid tissues and that the specific type of IF protein present is not related to the specific cell function: This is certainly a perplexing, negative statement; it also reminds us of the general question as to the biological functions of IFs and desmosomes, which is still unanswered.

Reticular Tissues with Specialized Epithelial Components
Various kinds of cells form meshwork (reticula) extending through the thymus and various parts of lymph nodes (Table 2). Some of these reticular cells are associated with a basal lamina, and others are not. In many of these cells (although not in all), cytokeratin IFs coexist with IFs containing other proteins, notably vimentin and/or desmin (Franke and Moll 1987), but subpopulations of thymic reticulum epithelium cells containing glial filament and neurofilament proteins have also been identified (see, e.g., Lee et al. 1988). A special form of such a reticular tissue is the meshwork of endothelium-type "stellate" cells, most but not all of which are positive for factor-VIII-related antigen(s). The cells constituting this meshwork, which traverses the lymph node sinus and is thus exposed within the vascular lumen, are connected by plaque-bearing junctions containing desmosomal proteins, in contrast to the monolayer of the general vascular lining endothelium.

155

Table 3 Examples of an Occurrence of Cytokeratins in Endothelia, Neurothelia, and Some Nonepithelial Tissues and Tumors of Certain Species

Mammals

A rare subtype of endothelial cells (e.g., in human synovia) (1)
All neurothelial cells of several species (see Table 1) (2)
Focally and irregularly in arachnoid cells of some species (3)
A subset of mesenchymal cells in human amniochorion and placenta (4)
Embryonal myocardium of some species (e.g., transient expression of cytokeratins 8 and 18 during human and chicken heart development) (5)
Smooth muscle cells of some fetal organs, notably blood vessels (6)
Focally and irregularly in some smooth muscle cells of adult tissues, notably myometrium, splenic trabeculae and atherosclerotic plaques, and in myomas and myosarcomas (7)
Focally and irregularly in certain subtypes of some nonepithelial tumors such as lymphomas, histiocytomas, melanomas, chondrosarcomas, pheochromocytomas, astrocytomas, gliosarcomas, and glioblastomas (8)

Amphibia (*Xenopus, Rana, Triturus*)

All endothelia (9)
All neurothelia (10)
Oocytes (11)
Certain types of smooth muscle (vascular, gastrointestinal) (12)
Blastema of regenerating limb (13)
Notochord (14)
Glial cells of optic nerve (15)
Ependymal cells (16)

Fish (rainbow trout) (17)

All endothelia, including pillar cells of gills
Scale-associated mesenchymal cells
Dermal fibroblasts
Certain types of vascular smooth muscle cells
Glial cells of optic nerve
Certain chondrocytes (15)

References: (1) Jahn et al. (1987); Franke et al. (1988). (2) Jahn et al. (1987); Ortonne et al. (1987); Ferretti et al. (1988); Achtstätter et al. (1989). (3) Theaker et al. (1986); Terpe et al. (1988); Achtstätter et al. (1989). (4) Khong et al. (1986). (5) Van Muijen et al. (1987); Kuruc and Franke (1988). (6) Jahn et al. (1987); Norton et al. (1987); Van Muijen et al. (1987); Bader et al. (1988); Kasper et al. (1988a). (7) Huitfeld and Brandtzaeg (1985); Bolen et al. (1986); Brown et al. (1987); Jahn et al. (1987); Norton et al. (1987); Van Muijen et al. (1987); Jahn and Franke (1989). (8) Sewell et al. (1986); Lawson et al. (1987); Perentes and Rubinstein (1987); Dervan et al. (1988); Hirose et al. (1988); Weiss et al. (1988). (9) Godsave et al. (1986); Jahn et al. (1987); Achtstätter et al. (1989). (10) Jahn et al. (1987); Ferretti et al. (1988); Achtstätter et al. (1989). (11) Franz et al. (1983). (12) Jahn et al. (1987). (13) Ferretti et al. (1988). (14) Godsave et al. (1986); LaFlamme et al. (1988); Herrmann et al. (1989). (15) Rungger-Brändle et al. (1988). (16) Godsave et al. (1986). (17) Markl and Franke (1988).

Cytokeratins and Desmosomes in Certain Nonepithelial Tissues
Cytokeratins have also been detected in several nonepithelial tissues (Table 3); in most cases, the specific cytokeratins identified are the simple epithelial cytokeratins 8 and 18 or their homologs in other species, occasionally together with some cytokeratin 19. Although the number of relevant studies in lower vertebrates is still very limited, it is already evident that cytokeratin expression in fish and amphibia is more widespread than that in higher vertebrates. For example, in these lower vertebrates, endothelia generally contain cytokeratin IFs (Jahn et al. 1987; Markl and Franke 1988). Of particular interest is the occurrence of large amounts of cytokeratin IFs in oocytes and eggs of certain species such as *Xenopus laevis*, as this maternal supply of cytokeratins apparently contributes to epithelial differentiation during early embryogenesis (Franz et al. 1983). It is also surprising that desmosomes and large amounts of cytokeratin IFs occur in a special type of astrocytes, i.e., those of the optic nerve glia of fish and amphibia (Markl and Franke 1988; Rungger-Brändle et al. 1988), and that cytokeratins are found in most (perhaps all) fibroblasts of fish dermis (Markl and Franke 1988).

Another remarkable finding is the occurrence of some cytokeratins in certain muscle tissue (Table 3), notably in smooth muscles of embryonal or fetal organs. Cytokeratins have also been seen in some normal adult smooth muscle tissues such as the myometrium, as well as in a percentage of myomas and myosarcomas, albeit only focally and to greatly variable extents. The synthesis of cytokeratins 8, 18, and 19 in smooth muscle cells has been studied in detail using human umbilical vessels, in which most of the smooth muscle cells are positive for cytokeratins by immunocytochemistry (see, e.g., Jahn et al. 1987; Van Muijen et al. 1987; Bader et al. 1988; Kasper et al. 1988a). However, quantitative determinations of cytokeratins present in this and other smooth muscle tissues have made it clear that the cytokeratins in these cells are present only in very low concentrations and represent only a miniscule proportion of the total IF protein present (Fig. 1 shows an analysis of a microdissected sample from an umbilical artery; for umbilical vein, see also Bader et al. 1988). The amounts of cytokeratins present in some adult smooth muscle tissues, such as myometrium and myomas in which cytokeratins are observed immunocytochemically much less consistently and usually only focally, are also very low (N. Kuruc and W.W. Franke, unpubl.).

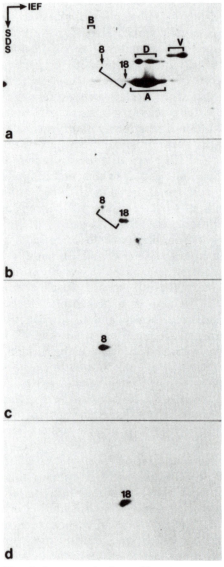

Figure 1 (*See facing page for legend.*)

Recent results from other laboratories are essentially in agreement with our findings (see, e.g., Van Muijen et al. 1987; Gown et al. 1988; Kasper et al. 1988a; Turley et al. 1988), although the specific mode of presentation chosen tends to result in an overestimation of the amounts of cytokeratins present in some of these reports. In our experience, smooth muscle cells containing cytokeratins occur with remarkable frequency in the vascular walls of human synovial tissue, especially in patients suffering from rheumatoid arthritis (Fig. 2a–e), and in human spleen (Fig. 2f,g) where such cells can also be found in avascular trabeculae (Fig. 3). Moreover, we have found that the frequency of cytokeratin-positive smooth muscle cells is often markedly increased in atherosclerotic plaques of human arterial biopsies (Jahn and Franke 1989).

The occurrence of cytokeratins in muscle cells, however, is not confined to smooth muscle tissues. Transient cytokeratin expression has been noted in myocardial tissue of human fetuses (cytokeratins 8 and 18) and chicken embryos (apparently only cytokeratin 8) but not in comparable developmental stages of several other vertebrate species (Van Muijen et al. 1987; Kuruc and Franke 1988). Of particular biological interest in this context is the recent study of Ferretti et al. (1988), who found that during new limb regeneration, cytokeratins 8 and 18 are transiently expressed in the mesenchymal blastema cells from which the various regenerating tissues, including striated muscle, will subsequently form.

Figure 1 Two-dimensional gel electrophoresis of residual proteins after extraction with buffer containing Triton X-100 from microdissected wall tissue of a human umbilical cord artery (for details and corresponding results obtained with vein wall tissue, see Bader et al. 1988). (IEF) Direction of isoelectric focusing; (SDS) direction of second-dimension electrophoresis in the presence of SDS. (a) Coomassie blue staining: (A) endogenous actin; (D) desmin; (V) vimentin; (B) bovine serum albumin added as reference protein; cytokeratins are numbered according to Moll et al. (1982). (b–d) Immunoblot reactions using different antibodies to cytokeratin polypeptides. Note that in a, actin, desmin, and vimentin are major cytoskeletal polypeptides, whereas cytokeratins are hardly detectable (bracket and arrows). In autoradiographs of immunoblots of preparations in parallel to the gel shown in a, cytokeratins 8 and 18 are detected, using monoclonal antibodies reacting either with a broad range of cytokeratin polypeptides (b, antibody K_G 8.13) or specifically with individual cytokeratin polypeptides (c, antibody K_S 8.1.42, specific for cytokeratin 8; d, antibody K_S 18.174, specific for cytokeratin 18).

Proteins immunologically cross-reactive with cytokeratins have also been seen, in some mammalian species, in neural structures apart from neurothelia and ependymal cells, such as special arrays in neuronal and glial elements (Masters et al. 1985; Franko et al. 1987). The biochemical significance of these isolated immunological observations is not clear.

Various investigators have reported immunolocalization of material cross-reactive with cytokeratins in tumors believed to be derived from nonepithelial cells (Table 3 includes some examples). However, in most of these studies, a positive reaction was seen only in some of the tumors, the distribution of the

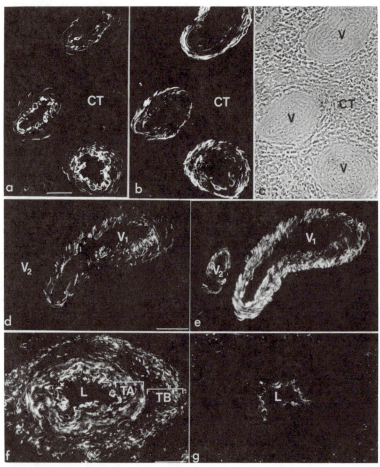

Figure 2 (*See facing page for legend.*)

160

cytokeratin-positive cells was focally restricted, and the immunostaining was often weak and sometimes appeared unusual, i.e., nonfibrillar. Clearly, experimental evidence from other methods is needed to substantiate such findings. Obviously, however, systematic studies of such inconsistent, low-level cytokeratin expression in variable focal patterns are very difficult.

Induction of Cytokeratin Synthesis in Cultured Cells

Typically, differentiated cells grown in vitro maintain the expression of many of the cytoskeletal proteins characteristic of the differentiated state of the tissue cells from which they are derived. In general, this holds for desmosomal and cytokeratins (see, e.g., Franke et al. 1979d, 1982b; Osborn and Weber 1983; Cowin et al. 1985a,b; Quinlan et al. 1985; Sun et al. 1985). However, examples of changes of synthesis of IF proteins during cell culturing have also been reported, particularly the additional synthesis of vimentin IFs, and some of these changes are obviously induced by the specific composition of the growth medium (see, e.g., Connell and Rheinwald 1983; Schmid et al. 1983; Sun et al. 1985; Kim et al. 1987). Even the complete cessation of cytokeratin synthesis, resulting in cells that contain only vimentin IFs or no IFs at all, has been described in some cultured cell lines and clones as, for example, in certain rat hepatoma cells (see, e.g., Venetianer et al. 1983).

Figure 2 Double-label immunofluorescence microscopy performed on sections of frozen synovial tissue from a patient suffering from rheumatoid arthritis (a–e; for details, see Jahn et al. 1987) and on cryostat sections of presumably unaltered spleen (f,g; for details, see Franke and Moll 1987). (a–e) Reactions of guinea pig antibodies against cytokeratins 8 and 18 (a,d) are compared with those of a murine monoclonal antibody to desmin (b,e), showing the location of these cytokeratins in some, but not all, smooth muscle cells of the vascular walls, in some places coexisting with desmin (c, phase-contrast micrograph corresponding to a and b). Typically, most cytokeratin-positive cells are located in the inner portions of the vascular walls, whereas cells rich in desmin are concentrated in abluminal regions. A vessel without any cytokeratin reaction is seen in d (V_2), next to a vessel with many cytokeratin-positive cells (V_1). The reaction of murine monoclonal antibody K_S 18.174 (f), in combination with that of rabbit antibodies to factor-VIII-related antigen (g) on a trabecular arteriole (TA) of spleen with associated trabecula (TB), reveals cytokeratin 18 expression in cells of the vascular wall, as well as in cells of the trabecula. The endothelial cells of this vessel, which are positive for factor VIII, are negative for cytokeratin 18. (L) Lumina; (CT) connective tissue. Bars, 50 μm.

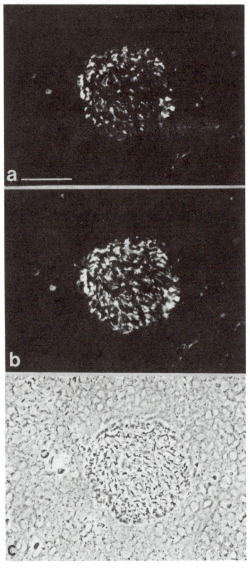

Figure 3 Double-label immunofluorescence microscopy of cryostat sections through human spleen tissue, using guinea pig antibodies to cytokeratins 8 and 18 (*a*), in combination with a murine monoclonal antibody to desmin (*b*). Intense cytokeratin reaction is seen, which is restricted to a subset of smooth muscle cells, whereas other smooth muscle cells within the trabecula show only weak or no reaction. The corresponding phase-contrast micrograph is shown in *c*. Bar, 50 μm.

The de novo appearance of cytokeratins and/or cytokeratin IFs in a cultured nonepithelium-derived cell is apparently a very rare event, except for the inducible synthesis of cytokeratins 8 and 18 in some cytokeratin-free pluripotent embryonal carcinoma cells (for references, see Franke and Moll 1987) or in cells derived from teratocarcinomas that resemble mesenchymal cells (Darmon et al. 1984; Darmon 1985; Sémat et al. 1986). This low frequency of cells starting cytokeratin synthesis spontaneously in culture may be surprising in view of the fact that such changes occur regularly during certain embryogenic processes, e.g., during the induction of kidney tubule formation from metanephric mesenchymal cells (see, e.g., Lehtonen et al. 1985). Nevertheless, the presence of cytokeratins in some cultured cells believed to be nonepithelial and nonpluripotent has been reported in several immunocytochemical studies, usually in low amounts (Trejdosiewicz et al. 1986; Zauli et al. 1986; for further references, see Franke and Moll 1987; Jahn et al. 1987; Kuruc and Franke 1988), although the specific cytokeratin polypeptides have not been unequivocally identified with biochemical methods.

Prompted by observations that individual cells or groups of cells immunochemically positive for cytokeratins 8 and 18 can be seen at low frequencies ($\sim 5 \cdot 10^{-4} - 10^{-6}$) in normally grown cultures of transformed human and rodent fibroblasts and other nonepithelial cells, we have recently studied the regulatory levels at which such changes take place. Therefore, we have selected cytokeratin-positive cells, enriched them in separate cultures, and compared them with the cytokeratin-negative cells from which they originated. By Northern blot and nuclear run-on analyses, we have shown that, for example, in most of the SV40-transformed human fibroblast lines examined, the gene(s) for cytokeratin 18 is actively transcribed, and translatable mRNA is accumulated. Moreover, low amounts of cytokeratin 18 are continually produced, but the resulting protein appears to be rapidly degraded and does not form stable IF structures so that these cells appear negative by immunocytochemistry. In contrast, the cells showing positive fibrillar immunostaining also contain considerable amounts of cytokeratin 8 mRNA and produce both cytokeratins 8 and 18 in considerable amounts. This indicates that the escape from the negative control of cytokeratin gene expression in such nonepithelial cells can take place in several steps and that a cell is usually only detected as cytokeratin-positive when the gene encoding cytokeratin 8 is also expressed. These observations, together with our finding that the vast majority of cells (≥90%) could be induced to form cytokeratin IFs by treatment with 5-azacytidine in some of these lines, suggest that the control of the genes encoding cytokeratins 8 and 18 (probably also 19) in these and probably other nonepithelial cells is not stringent and depends partially on stable CG methylation, in agreement with the results of Oshima et al. (1988) and Darmon and colleagues (Sémat et al. 1986).

CONCLUSIONS

Although true epithelial cells and the various types of epithelium-derived tumors are generally characterized by the constitutive formation of both cytokeratin IFs and desmosomes in all the diverse vertebrate species, the expression of these two classes of structures is not necessarily coupled in the layer-forming epithelioid tissues and in the reticulum-forming cell types, and marked differences can be observed between different vertebrate species. The reasons for these interspecies differences in junction formation and the specific composition of the IF cytoskeleton are not understood. In addition, we have learned that cytokeratins of the simple epithelium type, i.e., cytokeratins 8, 18, and 19, can appear in cells that are not organized in an epithelium, such as smooth muscle cells of certain species. Again, it is not understood why these cytokeratins are synthesized in certain subtypes of tissues, e.g., in some smooth muscles and not in others, and why such drastic differences exist between different species, different individuals of the same species, and different regions of the same organ. At present, we cannot decide whether the low-level cytokeratin synthesis observed in these nonepithelial cells defines distinct subsets of cells, merely reflects a tolerated "background synthesis" without any functional importance, or is due to positional or environmental influences.

Obviously, the possible occurrence of certain cytokeratins in some nonepithelial tissues and tumors—albeit irregularly, focally, and in low concentrations—has important implications for the immunocytochemical cell typing in practical tumor diagnosis. To improve the classification of the differentiated state of a given tumor and, hence, the diagnosis, a panel of antibodies to various marker proteins has to be used. Specifically, for the identification of epithelium-derived tumors such as carcinomas, the combined use of antibodies to both markers, cytokeratins and desmosomal proteins, is recommended. It will also be important to study whether the heterogeneity of cytokeratin expression in nonepithelial tissues and tumors is related to other biological differences in the cytokeratin-positive tissue regions and to examine whether these heterogeneities are related to possible selections of certain subforms from a complex tumor and to possible changes of the differentiation character during tumor growth, metastasis, and therapy.

REFERENCES

Achtstätter, T., B. Fouquet, E. Rungger-Brändle, and W.W. Franke. 1989. Cytokeratin filaments and desmosomes in the epithelioid cells of the perineural and arachnoidal sheaths of some vertebrate species. *Differentiation* (in press).

Achtstätter, T., R. Moll, A. Anderson, C. Kuhn, S. Pitz, K. Schwechheimer, and W.W. Franke. 1986. Expression of glial filament protein (GFP) in nerve sheaths and non-neural cells re-examined using monoclonal antibodies, with special emphasis on the coexpression of GFP and cytokeratins in epithelial cells of human salivary gland and pleomorphic adenomas. *Differentiation* 31: 206.

Alcala, J. and H. Maisel. 1985. Biochemistry of lens plasma membranes and cytoskeleton. In *The ocular lens* (ed. H. Maisel), p. 169. Marcel Dekker, New York.

Bader, B.L., L. Jahn, and W.W. Franke. 1988. Low level expression of cytokeratins 8, 18 and 19 in vascular smooth muscle cells of human umbilical cord and in cultured cells derived therefrom, with an analysis of the chromosomal locus containing the cytokeratin 19 gene. *Eur. J. Cell Biol.* 47: 300.

Barritault, D., Y. Courtois, and D. Paulin. 1980. Biochemical evidence that vimentin is the only in vivo constituent of the intermediate-sized filaments in adult bovine epithelial lens cells. *Biol. Cell* 39: 335.

Bolen, J.W., S.P. Hammar, and M.A. McNutt. 1986. Reactive and neoplastic serosal tissue: A light-microscopic, ultrastructural, and immunocytochemical study. *Am. J. Surg. Pathol.* 10: 34.

Brown, D.C., J.M. Theaker, P.M. Banks, K.C. Gatter, and D.Y. Mason. 1987. Cytokeratin expression in smooth muscle and smooth muscle tumours. *Histopathology* 11: 477.

Connell, N.D. and J.G. Rheinwald. 1983. Regulation of the cytoskeleton in mesothelial cells: Reversible loss of keratin and increase in vimentin during rapid growth in culture. *Cell* 34: 245.

Cooper, D. and T.-T. Sun. 1986. Monoclonal antibody analysis of bovine epithelial keratins. *J. Biol. Chem.* 261: 4646.

Cowin, P. and D.R. Garrod. 1983. Antibodies to epithelial desmosomes show wide tissue and species cross-reactivity. *Nature* 302: 148.

Cowin, P., H.-P. Kapprell, and W.W. Franke. 1985a. The complement of desmosomal plaque proteins in different cell types. *J. Cell Biol.* 101: 1441.

Cowin, P., W.W. Franke, C. Grund, H.-P. Kapprell, and J. Kartenbeck.

1985b. The desmosome-intermediate filament complex. In *The cell in contact* (ed. G. Edelman and J.P. Thiery), p. 427. Wiley, New York.

Czernobilsky, B., R. Moll, R. Levy, and W.W. Franke. 1985. Coexpression of cytokeratin and vimentin filaments in mesothelial, granulosa and *rete ovarii* cells of the human ovary. *Eur. J. Cell Biol.* **37:** 175.

Darmon, M. 1985. Coexpression of specific acid and basic cytokeratins in teratocarcinoma-derived fibroblasts treated with 5-azacytidine. *Dev. Biol.* **110:** 47.

Darmon, M., J.-F. Nicolas, and D. Lamblin. 1984. 5-Azacytidine is able to induce the conversion of teratocarcinoma-derived mesenchymal cells into epithelial cells. *EMBO J.* **3:** 961.

Dervan, P.A., J. O'Loughlin, and B.J. Hurson. 1988. Dedifferentiated chondrosarcoma with muscle and cytokeratin differentiation in the anaplastic component. *Histopathology* **12:** 517.

Docherty, R.J., J.G. Edwards, D.R. Garrod, and D.L. Mattey. 1984. Chick embryonic pigmented retina is one of the group of epithelioid tissues that lack cytokeratins and desmosomes and have intermediate filaments composed of vimentin. *J. Cell Sci.* **71:** 61.

Ferretti, P., D.M. Fekete, M. Patterson, and E.B. Lane. 1988. Keratin expression in undifferentiated mesenchymal cells of the regenerating newt limb. *Int. Congr. Cell Biol.* **4:** 147.

Franke, W.W. and R. Moll. 1987. Cytoskeletal components of lymphoid organs. I. Synthesis of cytokeratins 8 and 18 and desmin in subpopulations of extrafollicular reticulum cells of human lymph nodes, tonsils, and spleen. *Differentiation* **36:** 145.

Franke, W.W., C. Grund, and T. Achtstätter. 1986. Co-expression of cytokeratins and neurofilament proteins in a permanent cell line: Cultured rat PC12 cells combine neuronal and epithelial features. *J. Cell Biol.* **103:** 1933.

Franke, W.W., C. Grund, and E. Schmid. 1979a. Intermediate-sized filaments present in Sertoli cells are of the vimentin-type. *Eur. J. Cell Biol.* **19:** 269.

Franke, W.W., P. Cowin, M. Schmelz, and H.-P. Kapprell. 1987. The desmosomal plaque and the cytoskeleton. *Ciba Found. Symp.* **125:** 26.

Franke, W.W., E. Schmid, M. Osborn, and K. Weber. 1978a. Different intermediate-sized filaments distinguished by immunofluorescence microscopy. *Proc. Natl. Acad. Sci.* **75:** 5034.

———. 1979b. Intermediate-sized filaments of human endothelial cells. *J. Cell Biol.* **81:** 570.

Franke, W.W., E. Schmid, K. Weber, and M. Osborn. 1979c. HeLa cells contain intermediate-sized filaments of the prekeratin type. *Exp. Cell Res.* **118:** 95.

Franke, W.W., P. Cowin, C. Grund, C. Kuhn, and H.-P. Kapprell. 1988. The endothelial junction. The plaque and its components. In *Endothelial cell biology in health and disease* (ed. N. Simionescu and M. Simionescu), p. 147. Plenum Press, New York.

Franke, W.W., E. Schmid, S. Winter, M. Osborn, and K. Weber. 1979d. Widespread occurrence of intermediate-sized filaments of the vimentin-type in cultured cells from diverse vertebrates. *Exp. Cell*

Res. **123**: 25.

Franke, W.W., K. Weber, M. Osborn, R. Schmid, and C. Freudenstein. 1978b. Antibody to prekeratin. Decoration of tonofilament-like array in various cells of epithelial character. *Exp. Cell Res.* **116**: 429.

Franke, W.W., B. Appelhans, E. Schmid, C. Freudenstein, M. Osborn, and K. Weber. 1979e. Identification and characterization of epithelial cells in mammalian tissues by immunofluorescence microscopy using antibodies to prekeratin. *Differentiation* **15**: 1.

Franke, W.W., R. Moll, D.L. Schiller, E. Schmid, J. Kartenbeck, and H. Mueller. 1982a. Desmoplakins of epithelial and myocardial desmosomes are immunologically and biochemically related. *Differentiation* **23**: 115.

Franke, W.W., D.L. Schiller, R. Moll, S. Winter, E. Schmid, I. Engelbrecht, and H. Denk. 1981a. Diversity of cytokeratins. Differentiation specific expression of cytokeratin polypeptides in epithelial cells and tissues. *J. Mol. Biol.* **153**: 933.

Franke, W.W., E. Schmid, D. Breitkreutz, M. Lüder, P. Boukamp, N.E. Fusenig, M. Osborn, and K. Weber. 1979f. Simultaneous expression of two different types of intermediate-sized filaments in mouse keratinocytes proliferating *in vitro. Differentiation* **14**: 35.

Franke, W.W., E. Schmid, C. Grund, H. Mueller, I. Engelbrecht, R. Moll, J. Stadler, and E.-D. Jarasch. 1981b. Antibodies to high molecular weight polypeptides of desmosomes: Specific localization of a class of junctional proteins in cells and tissues. *Differentiation* **20**: 217.

Franke, W.W., E. Schmid, D.L. Schiller, S. Winter, E.-D. Jarasch, R. Moll, H. Denk, B. Jackson, and K. Illmensee. 1982b. Differentiation-related patterns of expression of proteins of intermediate-sized filaments in tissues and cultured cells. *Cold Spring Harbor Symp. Quant. Biol.* **46**: 431.

Franko, M.C., C.J. Gibbs, D.A. Rhoades, and D.C. Gajdusek. 1987. Monoclonal antibody analysis of keratin expression in the central nervous system. *Proc. Natl. Acad. Sci.* **84**: 3482.

Franz, J.K., L. Gall, M.A. Williams, B. Picheral, and W.W. Franke. 1983. Intermediate-size filaments in a germ cell: Expression of cytokeratins in oocytes and eggs of the frog *Xenopus. Proc. Natl. Acad. Sci.* **80**: 6254.

Fuchs, E., A.L. Tyner, G.J. Giudice, D. Marchuk, A.R. Chaudhury, and M. Rosenberg. 1987. The human keratin genes and their differential expression. *Curr. Top. Dev. Biol.* **22**: 5.

Fujimoto, T. and S.J. Singer. 1986. Immunocytochemical studies of endothelial cells in vivo. The presence of desmin only, or of desmin plus vimentin, or vimentin only, in the endothelial cells of different capillaries of the adult chicken. *J. Cell Biol.* **103**: 2775.

Giudice, G.J., S.M. Cohen, N.H. Patel, and M.S. Steinberg. 1984. Immunological comparison of desmosomal components from several bovine tissues. *J. Cell. Biochem.* **26**: 35.

Godsave, S.F., B.H. Anderton, and C.C. Wylie. 1986. The appearance and distribution of intermediate filament proteins during differentiation of the central nervous system, skin and notochord of *Xenopus laevis. J. Embryol. Exp. Morphol.* **97**: 201.

Gown, A.M., H.C. Boyd, Y. Chang, M. Ferguson, B. Reichler, and D.

Tippens. 1988. Smooth muscle cells can express cytokeratins of "simple epithelium." *Am. J. Pathol.* **132:** 223.

Granger, B.L. and E. Lazarides. 1984. Expression of the intermediate-filament-associated protein synemin in chicken lens cells. *Mol. Cell. Biol.* **4:** 1943.

Heid, H.W., I. Moll, and W.W. Franke. 1988. Patterns of expression of trichocytic and epithelial cytokeratins in mammalian tissues. II. Concomitant and mutually exclusive synthesis of trichocytic and epithelial cytokeratins in diverse human and bovine tissues (hair follicle, nail bed and matrix, lingual papilla, thymic reticulum). *Differentiation* **37:** 215.

Henzen-Logmans, S.C., H.V. Stel, G.N.P. Van Muijen, H. Mullink, and C.J.L.M. Meijer. 1988. Expression of intermediate filament proteins in adrenal cortex and related tumours. *Histopathology* **12:** 359.

Herrmann, H., B. Fouquet, and W.W. Franke. 1989. Expression of intermediate filament proteins during development of *Xenopus laevis*. I. cDNA clones encoding different forms of vimentin. *Development* **105:** (in press).

Hirose, T., T. Sano, A. Jun-ichi, and H. Kazuo. 1988. Malignant fibrous histiocytoma with epithelial differentiation? *Ultrastruct. Pathol.* **12:** 529.

Huitfeld, H.S. and P. Brandtzaeg. 1985. Various keratin antibodies produce immunohistochemical staining of human myocardium and myometrium. *Histochemistry* **83:** 381.

Jahn, L. and W.W. Franke. 1989. High frequency of cytokeratin-producing smooth muscle cells in human atherosclerotic plaques. *Differentiation* (in press).

Jahn, L., B. Fouquet, K. Rohe, and W.W. Franke. 1987. Cytokeratins in certain endothelial and smooth muscle cells of two taxonomically distant vertebrate species, *Xenopus laevis* and man. *Differentiation* **36:** 234.

Kapprell, H.-P., K. Owaribe, and W.W. Franke. 1988. Identification of a basic protein of M_r 75,000 as an accessory desmosomal plaque protein in stratified and complex epithelia. *J. Cell Biol.* **106:** 1679.

Kasper, M., R. Moll, and P. Stosiek. 1988a. Distribution of intermediate filaments in human umbilical cord: Unusual triple expression of cytokeratins, vimentin, and desmin. *Zool. Jahrb. Anat.* **117:** 227.

Kasper, M., R. Moll, P. Stosiek, and U. Karsten. 1988b. Patterns of cytokeratin and vimentin expression in the human eye. *Histochemistry* **89:** 369.

Kasper, M., R. Goertchen, P. Stosiek, G. Perry, and U. Karsten. 1986. Coexistence of cytokeratin, vimentin and neurofilament protein in human choroid plexus. An immunohistochemical study of intermediate filaments in neuroepithelial tissues. *Virchows Arch. A* **410:** 173.

Khong, T.Y., E.B. Lane, and W.B. Robertson. 1986. An immunocytochemical study of fetal cells at the maternal-placental interface using monoclonal antibodies to keratins, vimentin and desmin. *Cell Tissue Res.* **246:** 189.

Kim, K.H., V. Stellmach, J. Javors, and E. Fuchs. 1987. Regulation of human mesothelial cell differentiation: Opposing roles of retinoids and epidermal growth factor in the expression of intermediate filament proteins. *J. Cell Biol.* **105**: 3039.

Kuruc, N. and W.W. Franke. 1988. Transient coexpression of desmin and cytokeratins 8 and 18 in developing myocardial cells of some vertebrate species. *Differentiation* **38**: 177.

LaFlamme, S.E., M. Jamrich, L. Richter, T.D. Sargent, and I.B. Dawid. 1988. *Xenopus* endo B is a keratin preferentially expressed in the embryonic notochord. *Genes Dev.* **2**: 853.

LaRocca, P.J. and J.G. Rheinwald. 1984. Coexpression of simple epithelial keratins and vimentin by human mesothelium and mesothelioma in vivo and in culture. *Cancer Res.* **44**: 2991.

Laster, A.J., T. Itoh, T.J. Palker, and B.F. Haynes. 1986. The human thymic microenvironment: Thymic epithelium contains specific keratins associated with early and late stages of epidermal keratinocyte maturation. *Differentiation* **31**: 67.

Lawson, C.W., C. Fisher, and K.C. Gatter. 1987. An immunohistochemical study of differentiation in malignant fibrous histiocytoma. *Histopathology* **11**: 375.

Lee, I., B. Ochs, and W.W. Franke. 1988. Non-lymphoid parenchymal cells of the thymic medulla express all classes of intermediate filaments. *Lab. Invest.* **58**: 54A.

Lehtonen, E., I. Virtanen, and L. Saxén. 1985. Reorganization of intermediate filament cytoskeleton in induced metanephric mesenchyme cells is independent of tubule morphogenesis. *Dev. Biol.* **108**: 481.

Markl, J. and W.W. Franke. 1988. Localization of cytokeratins in tissues of the rainbow trout: Fundamental differences of expression patterns between fish and higher vertebrates. *Differentiation* **39**: 100.

Masters, C.L., B.L. McDonald, C. Lagenauer, M. Schachner, and M.C. Franke. 1985. Loop arrays in mouse brain demonstrated with antisera to cytokeratins and monoclonal antibodies to several classes of intermediate filaments: Strain differences and developmental expression. *Brain Res.* **334**: 267.

McKechnie, N.M., M. Boulton, H.L. Robey, F.J. Savage, and I. Grierson. 1988. The cytoskeleton elements of human retinal pigment epithelium: In vitro and in vivo. *J. Cell Sci.* **91**: 303.

Miettinen, M., R. Clark, and I. Virtanen. 1986. Intermediate filament proteins in choroid plexus and ependyma and their tumors. *Am. J. Pathol.* **123**: 231.

Moll, R., R. Krepler, and W.W. Franke. 1983. Complex cytokeratin polypeptide patterns observed in certain human carcinomas. *Differentiation* **23**: 256.

Moll, R., W.W. Franke, D.L. Schiller, B. Geiger, and R. Krepler. 1982. The catalog of human cytokeratin polypeptides: Patterns of expression of specific cytokeratins in normal epithelia, tumors and cultured cells. *Cell* **31**: 11.

Mueller, H. and W.W. Franke. 1983. Biochemical and immunological characterization of desmoplakins I and II, the major polypeptides of the desmosomal plaque. *J. Mol. Biol.* **163**: 647.

Norton, A.J., J.A. Thomas, and P.G. Isaacson. 1987. Cytokeratin-specific monoclonal antibodies are reactive with tumours of smooth muscle derivation. An immunocytochemical and biochemical study using antibodies to intermediate filament cytoskeletal proteins. *Histopathology* **11**: 487.

Ortonne, J.-P., P. Verrando, G. Pautrat, and M. Darmon. 1987. Lamellar cells of sensory receptors and perineural cells of nerve endings of pig skin contain cytokeratins. *Virchows Arch. A* **410**: 547.

Osborn, M. and K. Weber. 1983. Tumor diagnosis by intermediate filament typing: A novel tool for surgical pathology. *Lab. Invest.* **48**: 372.

Osborn, M., W.W. Franke, and K. Weber. 1980. Direct demonstration of the presence of two immunologically distinct intermediate sized filament systems in the same cell by double immunofluorescence microscopy. *Exp. Cell Res.* **125**: 37.

Oshima, R.G., K. Trevor, L.H. Shevinsky, O.A. Ryder, and G. Cecena. 1988. Identification of the gene coding for the endo B murine cytokeratin and its methylated, stable inactive state in mouse nonepithelial cells. *Genes Dev.* **2**: 505.

Owaribe, K., J. Kartenbeck, E. Rungger-Brändle, and W.W. Franke. 1988. Cytoskeletons of retinal pigment epithelial cells: Interspecies differences of expression patterns indicate independence of cell function from the specific complement of cytoskeletal proteins. *Cell Tissue Res.* **254**: 301.

Paranko, J., M. Kallajoki, L.J. Pelliniemi, V.-P. Lehto, and I. Virtanen. 1986. Transient coexpression of cytokeratin and vimentin in differentiating rat Sertoli cells. *Dev. Biol.* **117**: 35.

Peltonen, J., S. Jaakkola, I. Virtanen, and L. Pelliniemi. 1987. Perineurial cells in culture. An immunocytochemical and electron microscopic study. *Lab. Invest.* **57**: 480.

Perentes, E. and L.J. Rubinstein. 1987. Recent application of immunoperoxidase histochemistry in human neuro-oncology. *Arch. Pathol. Lab. Med.* **111**: 796.

Quinlan, R.A., D.L. Schiller, M. Hatzfeld, T. Achtstätter, R. Moll, J.L. Jorcano, T.M. Magin, and W.W. Franke. 1985. Patterns of expression and organization of cytokeratin intermediate filaments. *Ann. N.Y. Acad. Sci.* **455**: 282.

Ramaekers, F.C.S., M. Osborn, E. Schmid, K. Weber, H. Bloemendal, and W.W. Franke. 1980. Identification of the cytoskeletal proteins in lens forming cells, a special epithelioid cell type. *Exp. Cell Res.* **127**: 309.

Rungger-Brändle, E., T. Achtstätter, and W.W. Franke. 1988. Cytokeratins and desmosomal proteins in perineural epithelia and astroglia of amphibia. In *European Symposium on the Structure and Functions of the Cytoskeleton* (ed. B. Rousset), p. 105. IVth Meeting of the European Cytoskeletal Club, University of Lyon, France. INSERM 197.

Schiller, D.L., W.W. Franke, and B. Geiger. 1982. A subfamily of relatively large and basic cytokeratin polypeptides as defined by peptide mapping is represented by one or several polypeptides in epithelial cells. *EMBO J.* **1**: 761.

Schlegel, R., S. Banks-Schlegel, and G.S. Pinkus. 1980. Immunohistochemical localization of keratin in normal human tissues. *Lab. Invest.* **42**: 91.

Schmelz, M., R. Duden, P. Cowin, and W.W. Franke. 1986a. A constitutive transmembrane glycoprotein of M_r 165,000 (desmoglein) in epidermal and nonepidermal desmosomes. I. Biochemical identification of the polypeptide. *Eur. J. Cell Biol.* **42:** 177.

———. 1986b. A constitutive transmembrane glycoprotein of M_r 165,000 (desmoglein) in epidermal and nonepidermal desmosomes. II. Immunolocalization and microinjection studies. *Eur. J. Cell Biol.* **42:** 184.

Schmid, E., D.L. Schiller, C. Grund, J. Stadler, and W.W. Franke. 1983. Tissue type sepcific expression of intermediate filament proteins in a cultured epithelial cell line from bovine mammary gland. *J. Cell Biol.* **96:** 37.

Schmid, E., S. Tapscott, G.S. Bennett, J. Croop, S.A. Fellini, H. Holtzer, and W.W. Franke. 1979. Differential location of different types of intermediate-sized filaments in various tissues of the chick embryo. *Differentiation* **15:** 27.

Sémat, A., P. Duprey, M. Vasseur, and M. Darmon. 1986. Mesenchymal-epithelial conversions induced by 5-azacytidine: Appearance of cytokeratin endo-A messenger RNA. *Differentiation* **31:** 61.

Sewell, H.F., W.D. Thompson, and D.J. King. 1986. IgD myeloma/immunoblastic lymphoma cells expressing cytokeratin. *Br. J. Cancer* **53:** 695.

Steinberg, M.S., H. Shida, G.J. Giudice, M. Shida, N.H. Patel, and O.W. Blaschuk. 1987. On the molecular organization, diversity and functions of desmosomal proteins. *Ciba Found. Symp.* **125:** 3.

Steinert, P.M. and D.R. Roop. 1987. Molecular and cellular biology of intermediate filaments. *Annu. Rev. Biochem.* **57:** 593.

Sun, T.-T. and H. Green. 1978. Keratin filaments of cultured human epidermal cells. Formation of intermolecular disulfide bonds during terminal differentiation. *J. Biol. Chem.* **253:** 2053.

Sun, T.-T., C.H. Shih, and H. Green. 1979. Keratin cytoskeletons in epithelial cells: Growth, structural and antigenic properties. *Cell. Immunol.* **83:** 1.

Sun, T.-T., S.C.G. Tseng, A.J.-W. Huang, D. Cooper, A. Schermer, M.H. Lynch, R. Weiss, and R. Eichner. 1985. Monoclonal antibody studies of mammalian epithelial keratins: A review. *Ann. N.Y. Acad. Sci.* **455:** 307.

Terpe, H.-J., M. Kasper, H. Martin, and J. Lehmann. 1988. Nachweis von Cytokeratin in Zellen der Arachnoidea und in Meningiomen. *Zentralbl. Allg. Pathol. Pathol. Anat.* **134:** 259.

Theaker, J.M., K.C. Gatter, M.M. Esiri, and K.A. Fleming. 1986. Epithelial membrane antigen and cytokeratin expression by meningiomas: An immunohistological study. *J. Clin. Pathol.* **39:** 435.

Traub, P. 1985. *Intermediate filaments*. Springer-Verlag, Berlin.

Trejdosiewicz, L.K., J. Southgate, J.T. Kemshead, and G.M. Hodges. 1986. Phenotypic analysis of cultured melanoma cells. Expression of cytokeratin-type intermediate filaments by the M5 human melanoma cell line. *Exp. Cell Res.* **164:** 388.

Turley, H., K.A.F. Pulford, K.C. Gatter, and D.Y. Mason. 1988. Biochemical evidence that cytokeratins are present in smooth muscle. *Br. J. Exp. Pathol.* **69:** 433.

Van Muijen, G.N.P., D.J. Ruiter, and S.O. Warnaar. 1987. Coexpression of intermediate filament polypeptides in human fetal and adult tissues. *Lab. Invest.* **57:** 359.

Van Vorstenbosch, C.J.A.H.V., B. Colenbrander, C.J.G. Wensing, F.C.S. Raemakers, and G.P. Vooijs. 1984. Cytoplasmic filaments in fetal and neonatal pig testis. *Eur. J. Cell Biol.* **34:** 292.

Venetianer, A., D.L. Schiller, T. Magin, and W.W. Franke. 1983. Cessation of cytokeratin expression in a rat hepatoma cell line lacking differentiated functions. *Nature* **305:** 730.

Weiss, S.W., G.L. Bratthauer, and P.A. Morris. 1988. Postirradiation malignant fibrous histiocytoma expressing cytokeratin. Implications for the immunodiagnosis of sarcomas. *Am. J. Surg. Pathol.* **12:** 554.

Zauli, D., M. Gobbi, C. Crespi, P.L. Tazzari, F. Miserocchi, M. Magnani, and N. Testoni. 1986. Vimentin and keratin intermediate filaments expression by K562 leukemic cell line. *Leukemia Res.* **10:** 29.

Cytoskeletal and Cell-surface Markers of Embryonal Carcinomas and Teratocarcinomas

I. Damjanov, Y. Tani, R.K. Clark, S. Teshima, and A. Damjanov

Department of Pathology and Cell Biology
Jefferson Medical College of Thomas Jefferson University
Philadelphia, Pennsylvania 19107

As the name implies, human germ cell tumors originate from germ cells in the testis, ovary, or extragonadal sites. These tumors may be subdivided into several groups on the basis of their histological features, architectural complexity, and presumed histogenesis. However, irrespective of the classification used, in the testis it is important to distinguish seminomas, tumors of relatively good prognosis, from all other non-seminomatous germ cell tumors (NSGCT), which represent a distinct group of neoplasms, both clinically and biologically.

The histogenesis of human germ cell tumors and the relationship of seminomas to NSGCT have not been unequivocally established. Although it has been generally accepted that all of these tumors originate from the germ cell line, i.e., the spermatogenic and ovogenic cells, there is no consensus whether they originate from premeiotic primordial germ cells, from early spermatogonia and oogonia, or from postmeiotic cells. The stem cells of established tumors may have some resemblance to germ cells, such as in seminomas (dysgerminomas), but more often they assume features of embryonic cells (embryonal carcinoma), extraembryonic or fetal membranes (yolk sac carcinoma and choriocarcinoma), and even fetal or adult-like somatic cells (e.g., immature neural teratoma).

In view of the well-established germ cell derivation of germ cell tumors and the variable morphology of their stem cells, it was of interest to compare the cytoskeleton and cell-surface properties of various tumor cells and their presumptive progenitors, as well as the normal embryonic/extraembryonic and fetal cells to which they have been compared.

173

The human oocyte does not contain a fibrillar network of intermediate filaments, in contrast to the fibrillar network of *Xenopus laevis* (for review, see Lehtonen et al. 1988). Whether human oogenic cells contain the cytokeratin-like protein described in the mouse oocytes remains to be determined. The spermatogenic cells in the adult testis, like those in rodents, do not have detectable intermediate filaments, and it is not known whether their predecessors in the fetal gonads have any intermediate filaments either. Like the spermatogenic cells, the earliest form of malignancy in the testis, the so-called intratubular neoplasia or carcinoma in situ (Skakkebaek et al. 1987) does not contain an immunohistochemically detectable intermediate filament network.

Seminomas are typically devoid of intermediate filaments, although some cells stain with antibodies to vimentin and the tumor may sporadically contain cytokeratin-positive trophoblastic giant cells (Miettinen et al. 1985). Like fetal testicular germ cells, carcinoma in situ (CIS) and seminoma/dysgerminoma cells express placental alkaline phosphatase and the GL-7 globoseries carbohydrate antigen SSEA-3, defined by the monoclonal antibody raised to murine stage-specific embryonic antigen 3 (Andrews and Damjanov 1985). These cells have highly glycosylated membranes and express an array of lectin-binding oligosaccharide chains on their surface (Lee et al. 1985). The pattern of lectin binding is not pathognomonic and indicates that the glycosylation in these tumors occurs in a rather haphazard manner, retaining some similarity to carbohydrates on spermatogenic cells. These findings are consistent with the view that CIS and seminoma/dysgerminoma cells correspond to undifferentiated germ cells and thus differ from stem cells of other germ cell tumors, which have the phenotype of postmeiotic cells equivalent to cells normally found in the embryos and extra-embryonic membranes.

Embryonal carcinomas may be developmentally nullipotent and monomorphic or developmentally pluripotent. The latter cells assume the function of stem cells of teratocarcinomas, which are more commonly known as NSGCT in clinical parlance. Mixed germ cell tumors composed of seminomas and NSGCT account for 10–15% testicular tumors, indicating that both components could have a common cell of origin. CIS occurs in the seminiferous tubules of the testis involved by NSGCT and is immunohistochemically indistinguishable from CIS adjacent to seminomas, further implying a common developmental pathway for these germ cell tumors. However, in contrast to seminomas, embryonal carcinoma cells have a cytoskeleton that contains cytokeratin polypeptides. Western blot analysis of embryonal carcinoma stem cell lines cultured in vitro revealed 40-, 45-, and 52-kD cytokeratin polypeptides (Damjanov et al. 1984). Some cells also express vimentin filaments. Embryonal carcinoma cells express the carbohydrate antigens recognized by the antibodies to the mouse SSEA-3 and SSEA-4 and are also rich in alkaline phosphatase (Andrews and Damjanov 1985). In this respect, the human embryonal carcinoma cells differ from equivalent mouse cells, which apparently do not contain cytokeratin filaments and express the lactoseries rather than the globoseries antigens found on human embryonal carcinoma cells.

It has not been definitively established whether all human embryonal carcinoma cells have a cytoskeleton rich in cytokeratin filaments. Studies on the newly established pluripotent stem cell line NCCIT (Teshima et al. 1988) suggest that the pluripotent stem cells do not have a filamentous network of cytokeratin but develop it soon after differentiation into morphologically distinct descendants. It would thus appear that the stem cells of human embryonal carcinoma cells vary from one case to another and correspond to embryonic cells at various stages of development. Therefore, according to their differentiation, these cells might or might not have cytokeratin filaments. However, it appears that most, if not all, embryonal carcinoma cells differentiate spontaneously into cytokeratin-positive descendants, which are readily detectable in histologic sections of surgically removed solid tumors. This may be used in surgical pathology for evaluation of germ cell tumors and for distinguishing seminomas from embryonal carcinoma (Battifora et al. 1984).

In contrast to embryonal carcinoma stem cells that correspond to cells of the embryo proper, choriocarcinoma cell lines are equivalent to cytotrophoblastic and syncytiotrophoblastic cells of the placenta. Like the normal chorionic cells, these cells secrete chorionic gonadotropin and other placental proteins and express the typical placental isoenzyme of the alkaline phosphatase (Andrews and Damjanov 1985). Like the cytoskeleton of the normal trophoblast, the cytoskeleton of these cells consists of 40-, 45-, 52-, and 54-kD (nos. 19, 18, 8, and 7) cytokeratin polypeptides (Clark and Damjanov 1985). The 54-kD cytokeratin polypeptide could thus serve as a marker for trophoblastic differentiation in human germ cell tumors.

Mouse trophoectodermal carcinoma cell line E6496D (Damjanov et al. 1985) also has a cytokeratin-rich cytoskeleton which, like the placenta in vivo, contains the mouse equivalents of human keratins (nos. 19, 18, 8, and 7). In contrast, like normal yolk sac in utero, yolk sac cell lines express only cytokeratin numbers 19, 18, and 8. Thus, by analogy with human germ cell tumors, cytokeratin number 7 appears to be a marker for trophectodermal differentiation.

In summary, antibodies to cytokeratin polypeptides are useful reagents for diagnosis and evaluation of human, as well as murine, germ cell tumors.

REFERENCES
Andrews, P.W. and I. Damjanov. 1985. Immunohistochemistry of human teratocarcinoma stem cells. In *Monoclonal antibodies and cancer* (ed. S. Sell and R.A. Reisfeld), p. 339. Humana Press, Clifton, New Jersey.
Battifora, H., K. Sheibani, R. Tubbs, M.I. Kopinsky, and T.T. Sun. 1984. Antikeratin antibodies in tumor diagnosis. Distinction between seminoma and embryonal carcinoma. *Cancer* **54:** 843.
Clark, R.K. and I. Damjanov. 1985. Intermediate filaments of human trophoblast and choriocarcinoma cell lines. *Virchows Arch. Pathol. Anat.* **407:** 203.
Damjanov, I., R.K. Clark, and P.W. Andrews. 1984. Cytoskeleton of human embryonal carcinoma cells. *Cell Differ.* **15:** 133.
Damjanov, I., A. Damjanov, and P.W. Andrews. 1985. Trophectodermal carcinoma: Mouse teratocarcinoma derived tumour stem cell differentiating into trophoblastic and yolk sac elements. *J. Embryol. Exp. Morphol.* **86:** 125.
Lee, M.-C., A. Talerman, J.W. Oosterhuis, and I. Damjanov. 1985. Lectin histochemistry of classical and spermatocytic seminoma. *Arch. Pathol. Lab. Med.* **109:** 938.
Lehtonen, E., G. Ordonez, and I. Reima. 1988. Cytoskeleton in preimplantation mouse development. *Cell. Differ.* **24:** 165.
Miettinen, M., I. Virtanen, and A. Talerman. 1985. Intermediate filament proteins in human testis and testicular germ cell tumors. *Am. J. Pathol.* **120:** 402.
Skakkebaek, N.E., J.G. Berthelsen, A. Giwercman, and J. Miller. 1987. Carcinoma-in-situ of the testis: Possible origin from gonocytes and precursor of all types of germ cell tumours except spermatocytoma. *Int. J. Androl.* **10:** 19.
Teshima, S., Y. Shimosato, S. Hirohashi, Y. Tome, I, Hayashi, H. Kanazawa, and T. Kakizoe. 1988. Four new human germ cell tumor lines. *Lab. Invest.* **59:** 328.

Expression of Intermediate Filaments in Developing Tissues and Cultured Cells

I. Virtanen, M. Hormia, M. Järvinen, T. Kivelä, and L. Laitinen

Departments of Anatomy and Ophthalmology, University of Helsinki
SF-00170 Helsinki, Finland

Expression of Intermediate Filaments in Developing Tissues and Tumors

The major cell types in human tissues express intermediate filaments (IFs) in a cell-type-specific manner, in line with our view on the histogenetic origin of different cell types: Vimentin is found in mesenchymal cells, desmin in muscle cells, cytokeratins in epithelial cells, glial fibrillary acidic protein (GFAP) in astrocytes, and neurofilament proteins in neuronal cells (Virtanen et al. 1985; Steinert and Roop 1988). However, many studies have revealed that the patterns of expression of IFs may be much more complex during development.

Kidney tubular epithelial cells, although developing from the kidney mesenchyme, appear to acquire expression of cytokeratins and lose the expression of vimentin during tubulogenesis. This can also be induced in vitro (Lehtonen et al. 1985), suggesting that epithelial differentiation does not necessarily require tubule morphogenesis with its complex cell-to-cell interactions. Early studies on the expression of IFs in normal and tumor cells in vivo and in vitro concluded that most cells only express one type of IF (see, e.g., Virtanen et al. 1981, 1985). However, vimentin, in particular, is often coexpressed with the cell-type-specific IF protein. Such is the case with most cultured cells that usually contain vimentin (Virtanen et al. 1981). In addition, during embryonal development, some epithelial cells, as well as neuronal cells, may display vimentin immunoreactivity not found in the corresponding cells in adult tissues. Such transient coexpression of two types of IFs may even lead to the establishment of an unexpected IF pattern in adult cells: Sertoli cells in both adult rat and man contain only vimentin IFs (Virtanen et al. 1986), although they are of epithelial origin. During embryonic development, the Sertoli cells in both species contain cytokeratins 8 and 18, which disappear abruptly during hormonal maturation of the testis (Paranko et al. 1986). Such a dual expression of IFs during histogenesis may explain why Sertoli cell-like tumors, e.g., the tubular androblastomas, are cytokeratin immunoreactive.

Coexpression of vimentin and cytokeratins is a frequent observation in carcinomas, e.g., in thyroid, lung, and renal carcinomas (Virtanen et al. 1985). In some instances, such a dual expression may be of diagnostic significance, e.g., in the case of endometrial carcinomas, because other adenocarcinomas of differential diagnostic significance are usually devoid of vimentin immunoreactivity. Ramaekers et al. (1983) have suggested that coexpression of vimentin and cytokeratin IFs might be a typical feature of all metastatic carcinoma cells and could be due to aberrant gene expression caused by loss of normal cell-to-cell connections. Such a suggestion is supported by studies on cultured cells, as well as on some epithelial cells in embryonic tissues, such as the fetal rat genital ducts (Paranko and Virtanen 1986) and the stellate reticulum cells of early embryonic tooth germ. Our own results on large materials of carcinomas, however, suggest that carcinoma cells in metastases only rarely express vimentin immunoreactivity. Furthermore, thyroid adenomas, neoplasms that display both abundant desmosomes and adherent junctions, consistently express vimentin, together with cytokeratins.

There are also other examples of coexpression of two or even three types of IFs in normal and malignant cells. Cytokeratins and neurofilament proteins are often coexpressed in many, but not in all, neuroendocrine tumors (Virtanen et al. 1985). Examples of immunoreactive tumors are lung carcinoid tumors, islet cell tumors, and thyroid medullary carcinomas.

Expression of IF Cultured Cells

The examples mentioned in the previous section clearly show that IF expression in both developing and tumor cells may be controlled by mechanisms leading to patterns of expression that cannot be fully explained on the basis of the concept of tissue-specific IF expression. Such changes may suggest gene regulation mechanisms in which the IF pattern is more dependent on the state of the differentiation of the tumor cells than on their derivation.

The pattern of IF expression can give important information

about the origin and developmental history of cultured cells. Thus, the expression of cytokeratins or desmin in cultured cells strongly speaks in favor of their derivation from epithelial tissue or carcinoma or from muscle tissue or rhabdomyosarcoma, respectively. However, several examples illustrate the complexity of such an analysis: Venetianer et al. (1983) described that cultured hepatoma cells may lose IF expression completely. Similarly, mesothelial cells may also lose IF expression and cytokeratins may disappear and emerge again, depending on the culture conditions. In some cases, IF analysis may make it necessary to reevaluate the derivation of some widely used cell lines. This is exemplified by findings on PC12 pheochromocytoma cells, thought to be derived from a transplantable pheochromocytoma. They were recently shown to coexpress neurofilaments and cytokeratins (Franke et al. 1986). This finding would suggest that PC12 cells represent neuroendocrine cells, rather than neuronal cells.

In addition, IF expression in mesenchymal cells appears to be more complex than anticipated. Recently, we showed that if cultured in a complex medium, fetal, but not adult, human fibroblasts can be induced to express cytokeratins 8 and 18 (von Koskull and Virtanen 1987). Coexpression of cytokeratins, together with vimentin, also appears to be a common property of human fibrosarcoma cell lines, as it is also often seen in some mesenchymal tumors (Virtanen et al. 1985). Furthermore, in fibrosarcoma cells, cytokeratin immunoreactivity increased upon exposure to sodium butyrate but disappeared when exposed to a tumor-promoting phorbol ester. K562 erythroleukemia cells, capable of erythroid differentiation, were similarly shown to express cytokeratins 8, 18, and 19, together with vimentin (M. Järvinen et al., in prep.). In this cell line, the cytokeratin immunoreactivity disappeared upon erythroid differentiation but was substantially increased when exposed to the phorbol ester. These results suggest that the regulation of IF expression in cultured cells is a complex phenomenon, with different cell lines responding differently to various modulating agents. Furthermore, little is still known about the role of post-transitional modifications in the regulation of IF expression and function. In this respect, it is of interest that normal and malignant human mesenchymal cells appear to differ in their state of phosphorylation, as well as susceptibility to the action of Ca^{++}-activated protease (Virtanen et al. 1988a). Such differences in the phosphorylation status of neurofilament polypeptides, in particular, are also seen in normal tissues (Lee et al. 1987).

In the characterization of retinoblastomas and small cell carcinomas of the lung, great effort has been devoted to cell-culture studies to elucidate new features of their histogenesis and differentiation. First, in vivo studies on retinoblastomas implied that these tumors would be able to differentiate into glial-resembling cells. On the other hand, experiments with Y79 retinoblastoma cells in numerous studies have suggested that these cells are able to coexpress glial and neuronal markers, although such features have not been found in surgically removed retinoblastomas (Kivelä et al. 1986). Our recent results on Y79 retinoblastoma cells (Virtanen et al. 1988b) showed that the previous suggestions on their dual capability to differentiate may be due to cross-reaction of the polyclonal GFAP antibodies used in those studies. The results with a panel of neurofilament antibodies revealed that during dibutyryl cAMP-induced differentiation of Y79 cells on laminin-coated growth substratum, the cells acquired neuronal characteristics by their expression of phosphorylated neurofilaments but did not show GFAP immunoreactivity under any culture conditions. However, when plated on fibronect'n-coated growth substratum, the cells rapidly began to express cytokeratins 8 and 18, but not 19, resembling pigmented retinal epithelial cells, in this respect.

Neurofilament expression in small cell carcinomas of the lung has also been a topic of intense study (Virtanen et al. 1985). Most studies have failed to reveal neurofilament positivity in typical small cell carcinomas of the lung. Results with cultured cells, however, have shown that distinct cell lines derived from small cell carcinomas of the lung constitutively express neurofilaments and lack cytokeratins, suggesting that cells derived from these tumors are able to acquire and maintain neuronal differentiation.

ACKNOWLEDGMENTS

This study was supported by grants from the Finnish Cancer Research Fund, the Sigrid Juselius Foundation, and the Paulo Foundation and by a research contract with the Finnish Academy of Sciences.

REFERENCES
Franke, W.W., C. Grund, and T. Achtstätter. 1986 Co-expression of cytokeratal and neurofilament proteins in a permanent cell line:

Cultured rat PC12 cells combine neuronal and epithelial features. *J. Cell Biol.* **103:** 1933.

Kivelä, T., A. Tarkkanen, and I. Virtanen. 1986. Intermediate filaments in the human retina and retinoblastoma. *Invest. Ophthalmol. Visual Sci.* **27:** 1075.

Lee, V.M.-Y., M.J. Garden, W.W. Schlaepfer, and J.Q. Trojanowski. 1987. Monoclonal antibodies distinguish several differentially phosphorylated states of the two largest rat neurofilament subunits (NF-H and NF-M) and demonstrate their existence in the normal nervous system. *J. Neurosci.* **7:** 3474.

Lehtonen, E., I. Virtanen, and L. Saxén. 1985. Reorganization of intermediate filament cytoskeleton in induced metanephric mesenchyme cells is independent of tubule morphogenesis. *Dev. Biol.* **108:** 481.

Paranko, J. and I. Virtanen. 1986. Epithelial and mesenchymal cell differentiation in the fetal rat genital ducts: Changes in the expression of cytokeratin and vimentin type of intermediate filaments and desmosomal plaque proteins. *Dev. Biol.* **117:** 135.

Paranko, J., M. Kallajoki, L.J. Pelliniemi, V.-P. Lehto, and I. Virtanen. 1986. Transient coexpression of cytokeratin and vimentin in differentiating rat Sertoli cells. *Dev. Biol.* **117:** 35.

Ramaekers, F.C.S., D. Haag, A. Kant, O. Moesker, P.H.K. Jap, and G.P. Vooijs. 1983. Coexpression of keratin- and vimentin-type intermediate filaments in human metastatic carcinoma cells. *Proc. Natl. Acad. Sci.* **80:** 2618.

Steinert, P.M. and D.R. Roop. 1988. Molecular and cellular biology of intermediate filaments. *Annu. Rev. Biochem.* **57:** 593.

Venetianer, A., D.L. Schiller, T. Magin, and W.W. Franke. 1983. Cessation of cytokeratin expression in a rat hepatoma cell line lacking differentiated functions. *Nature* **305:** 730.

Virtanen, I., O. Närvänen, and V.-P. Lehto. 1988a. Differential immunoreactivity and Ca^{2+}-dependent degradation of vimentin in human fibroblasts and fibrosarcoma cells. *Int. J. Cancer* **42:** 256.

Virtanen, I., M. Miettinen, V.-P. Lehto, A.-L. Kariniemi, and R. Paasivuo. 1985. Diagnostic application of monoclonal antibodies to intermediate filaments. *Ann. N.Y. Acad. Sci.* **455:** 635.

Virtanen, I., M. Kallajoki, O. Närvänen, J. Paranko, L.-E. Thornell, M. Miettinen, and V.-P. Lehto. 1986. Peritubular myoid cells of human and rat testis are smooth muscle cells that contain desmin-type intermediate filaments. *Anat. Rec.* **215:** 10.

Virtanen, I., T. Kivelä, M. Bugnoli, C. Mencarelli, V. Pallini, D.M. Albert, and A. Taibbanen. 1988b. Expression of intermediate filaments and synaptophysin show neuronal properties and lack of glial characteristics in Y79 retinoblastoma cells. *Lab. Invest.* **59:** 649.

Virtanen, I., V.-P. Lehto, E. Lehtonen, T. Vartio, S. Stenman, P. Kurki, O. Wager, J.V. Small, D. Dahl, and R.A. Badley. 1981. Expression of intermediate filaments in cultured cells. *J. Cell Sci.* **50:** 45.

von Koskull, H. and I. Virtanen. 1987. Induction of cytokeratin expression in human mesenchymal cells. *J. Cell. Physiol.* **133:** 321.

Intercellular Adhering Junctions as Molecular Markers in Tumor Diagnosis

P. Cowin

Departments of Cell Biology and Dermatology
New York University Medical School, New York, New York 10016

Intercellular *Adhaerens* junctions are membrane domains structurally and biochemically specialized to form strong intercellular adhesions and to anchor several types of filaments. There are two major types: the desmosome (*macula adhaerens*) and the intermediate junctions (*fascia, zonula* and *punta adhaerens,* endothelial, lens, and sertoli cell junctions) (Farquhar and Palade 1963). Desmosomes link the intermediate filament (IF) cytoskeletons of neighboring cells, so "bracing" a tissue against mechanical stress. Intermediate junctions anchor actin filaments to form a contractile system throughout the tissue, which can produce dramatic alterations in tissue shape. Desmosomes are found in all epithelia, in meningial tissue, in cardiac-intercalated discs, and between the dendritic cells of lymph nodes (Cowin et al. 1985b). As a consequence, they are often used as markers of epithelial differentiation in the diagnosis of carcinomas (Moll et al. 1986) and, more recently, of meningiomas (Parrish et al. 1986). Intermediate junctions have a far broader distribution than desmosomes and are often confused with them because of their structural resemblance. This has presented a problem to the use of desmosomes as epithelial markers, which, however, can be overcome by means of antibodies to junction-specific molecules (Cowin et al. 1985a). Here, we review the current knowledge of each junctional component and indicate the practical applications of antibodies directed to them for pathology.

Desmosomes

The desmosome is composed of seven major components (Gorbsky and Steinberg 1981) (see Fig. 1).

Desmoplakins I and II. These components (250 and 215 kD, respectively) are found toward the cytoplasmic face of the desmosomal plaque (Miller et al. 1987). Their location and high

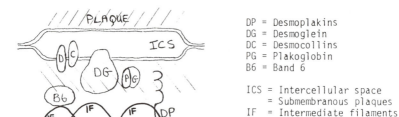

DP = Desmoplakins
DG = Desmoglein
DC = Desmocollins
PG = Plakoglobin
B6 = Band 6

ICS = Intercellular space
    = Submembranous plaques
IF = Intermediate filaments

Figure 1 Diagram of the relative positions of desmosomal proteins.

glycine content, a property that they share with the IF bundling protein filaggrin, suggest that they may function to bind the IF to the plaque (Cowin et al. 1985a). Desmoplakins I and II are closely related proteins (Muller et al. 1983; Cowin et al. 1985a), encoded by two mRNAs of 7 and 9 kb, which are transcribed from a single gene (Green et al. 1988). Our partial cDNA sequence shows six prominent GRSR (glycine, arginine, serine, arginine) repeats in the carboxyl terminus and regions of α-helicity (P. Cowin and W.W. Franke, unpubl.). Desmoplakin I is found in all desmosome plaques, whereas desmoplakin II is found only among cells derived from stratified tissues (Cowin et al. 1985a). Desmoplakins exist not only in a plasma-membrane-bound form, but also as a soluble cytoplasmic pool and as an insoluble cytosolic complex (Duden and Franke 1988; Pasdar and Nelson 1988a). There is considerable dispute as to whether the latter consists of membrane-bound endocytosed desmosomal remnants (Duden and Franke 1988) or as desmoplakin-IF complexes awaiting recruitment to the plasma membrane (Jones and Goldman 1985; Pasdar and Nelson 1988b). Monoclonal antibodies to desmoplakins have proven the most reliable markers of desmosomes and can be used to detect most types of carcinoma and meningioma (Moll et al. 1986; Parrish et al. 1986). The distinctive punctate fluorescent appearance of the antibody reaction can reliably detect micrometastases.

Plakoglobin. Plakoglobin (83 kD) was originally described as a component of the desmosomal plaque (Gorbsky et al. 1985). However, we have shown in more systematic Northern and Western analyses that plakoglobin and its mRNA are expressed not only in cells and tissues forming desmosomes, but also in those containing many types of intermediate junctions. It is found in a plaque-bound form and as a cytosolic dimer

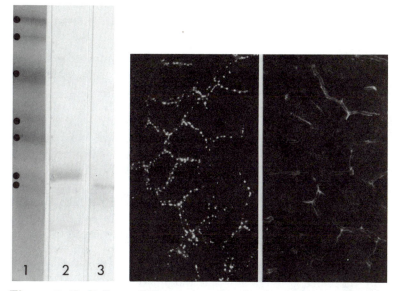

Figure 2 (*Left*) (Lane *1*) Desmosome fraction from bovine epidermis. Dots denote (from *top* to *bottom*) desmoplakin I, desmoplakin II, desmoglein, desmocollin I, desmocollin II, plakoglobin, and 76-kb band 6 protein.   Western blot reaction of monoclonal antibodies (lane *2*), plakoglobin (lane *3*), and 76-kb protein. (*Right*) 5-μm frozen sections of bovine liver stained with antibodies to desmoplakin (*left*; note the punctate appearance of desmosomes along the bile canaliculi) and to the 76-kd protein (*right*; note the linear straining of the zonular intermediate junction surrounding the bile canaliculi).

(Cowin et al. 1987). The localization of plakoglobin at these structurally similar, but otherwise biochemically diverse, junctional domains suggests that it plays a central role in the basic structure and function of symmetrically formed plaques, probably by interacting with the transmembrane components. Antibodies to this protein are of limited diagnostic use, as they recognize both classes of *adhaerens* junctions.

Band 6 protein. Band 6 protein is extremely basic (PI 8.0) and is detected only in stratified and complex epithelia (Kapprell et al. 1988). It can bind certain acidic cytokeratins in protein overlay techniques (Kapprell et al. 1988). Currently, no monoclonal antibodies are available for this desmosomal protein. Monoclonal antibodies to proteins that comigrate to the same position on SDS-polyacrylamide gels are described in Figure 2a; however, they locate to intermediate junctions found surrounding the bile canaliculi of liver (see Fig. 2b), between the cells surrounding kidney tubules, and in apical rings in cultured polarized cells.

Desmoglein. A calcium-binding transmembrane glycoprotein, desmoglein (165 kD) is found in all desmosomes (Schmelz et al. 1986a,b; Steinberg et al. 1987). It has been strongly implicated as the cell-surface antigen detected by pathogenic autoantibodies of the blistering disease *pemphigus foliaceus* (Eyre and Stanley 1987), suggesting that it plays a key role in the adhesive mechanism; 50 kD of desmoglein is exposed at the surface in stratified tissues and has both N- and O-linked glycosylation, but only the N-linked form is found in simple epithelia (Penn et al. 1988). A large, highly conserved domain of this protein lies on the cytoplasmic side of the cell membrane and contributes significantly to the plaque structure (Schmelz et al. 1986a,b). Monoclonal antibodies directed against these internal epitopes recognize this component in all desmosomes and therefore provide reliable diagnostic markers of desmosome-bearing tumors. Many antibodies, however, are restricted to stratified tissues (Cohen et al. 1983; Giudice et al. 1984), a feature that may reflect the tissue differences in the glycosylation.

Desmocollins I and II. These components (130 and 115 kD, respectively) have been localized to the intercellular space (Miller et al. 1987) and are expressed on the surface of cultured cells prior to cell contact or desmosome formation (Cowin et al. 1984). Cell types, derived from simple epithelia, modulate the distribution of their desmocollins to their basolateral surfaces at confluence, whereas cells that stratify in vitro continue to express them apically. Furthermore, addition of univalent desmocollin antibodies to the culture medium will inhibit desmosome assembly in vitro (Cowin et al. 1984). Taken together, our data strongly imply a central role for desmocollins in the initiation of desmosome assembly. Desmocollins I and II are biochemically and immunologically closely related (Muller and Franke 1983). They differ in size prior to glycosylation, as well as in their degree of glycosylation, and are not derived from one another (Kapprell et al. 1985; Penn et al. 1987). They are phosphorylated, bind calcium (Penn et al. 1987), and show tissue variation in their reaction with antibodies (Cowin and Garrod 1983). Whether this variability relates to tissue-specific modulation of adhesion is yet to be established, but in this context, it should be noted that desmosomes readily form between different cell types, suggesting that their adhesive components are compatible and do not contribute in a qualitative way to recognition (Mattey and Garrod 1985). Antisera to desmocollins have been applied to the diagnosis of meningiomas (Parrish et al. 1986). A further investigation is required to test whether the restricted tissue pattern of the monoclonal antibodies can be applied to a finer "fingerprinting" of the epithelial tissue of origin of certain tumors.

Minor Components of the Desmosome

Several minor components of the epidermal desmosomes have been described. However, their immunohistochemistry is presently incomplete; therefore, the capabilities of antibodies available to them as diagnostic aids remain uncertain. These include desmocalmin (240 kD), a calmodulin-binding plaque constituent that can bind to IFs in vitro in the presence of magnesium ions (Tsukita and Tsukita 1985); a 125-kD protein showing immunological reaction with E-cadherin antibodies (Jones 1988) and a 140-kD glycoprotein recognized by pemphigus sera (Jones et al. 1986), both of which are found not only within the desmosome, but also in the interdesmosomal membrane regions; and a 22-kD component of the desmoglea found in snout desmosomal preparations (Gorbsky and Steinberg 1981).

Intermediate Junctions

At the present time, no biochemical isolation procedures are available for intermediate junctions, and so our knowledge of their composition is incomplete. However, a number of components are known largely from the work of B. Geiger and colleagues (unpubl.), who have applied the powerful approach provided by monoclonal antibodies to the description of this set of junctions.

All intermediate junctions contain two components: vinculin (130 kD) plaque component (Ungar et al. 1986) and plakoglobin (83 kD) (Cowin et al. 1987). By virtue of their association to actin filaments, they are also enriched in actin-binding proteins, tropomyosin, and α-actinin (Ungar et al. 1986). In addition, two calcium-dependent adhesion molecules have been described: L-CAM (N-cadherin, uvomorulin; 120 kD) has been found in a variety of intermediate junctions of stratified and simple epithelia; A-CAM (135 kD) is absent from these junctions but present on intermediate junctions of lens, brain, cardiac muscle, and cultured kidney cells. Despite their different tissue distributions, heterotypic intermediate junctions can form in vitro between L-CAM containing liver cells and A-CAM containing lens cells, suggesting that these molecules may share significant functional homology (Volk et al. 1987).

Recently, a number of components have been described at various subsets of intermediate junctions, i.e., ZAITJ component (Kapprell et al. 1988), a 76-kD component (see Fig. 2), and an 82-kD protein (Tsukita and Tsukita 1988). However, the immunohistochemistry of these molecules is incomplete.

SUMMARY

From the immunohistochemical perspective, junctional molecules fall into three categories. (1) Those that are exclusive to, but present on, all desmosomes *or* intermediate junctions. Antibodies to these proteins, for example, desmoplakins, vinculin, and certain desmoglein antibodies, are extremely useful markers of their particular junction and, hence, of a particular differentiation pathway. These may have important uses for the diagnosis of carcinoma versus sarcoma. (2) Proteins that are common to both types of junction, e.g., plakoglobin and L-CAM. These have little diagnostic potential at the present time. (3) Proteins that are exclusive to desmosomes *or* intermediate junctions and furthermore recognize a subset within these types. The severe tissue restriction of many monoclonal antibodies to desmocollins may provide a very sensitive means to "fingerprint" the origin of tumors to a particular epithelial type or to recognize changes from a simple to a stratified epithelial phenotype, which accompany certain invasive states, e.g., cervical carcinoma.

REFERENCES

Cohen, S.M., G. Gorbsky, and M.S. Steinberg. 1983. Immunochemical characterization of related families of glycoproteins in desmosomes. *J. Biol. Chem.* **258:** 2621.

Cowin, P. and D.R. Garrod. 1983. Antibodies to epithelial desmosomes show wide tissue and species cross-reactivity. *Nature* **302:** 148.

Cowin, P., H.-P. Kapprell, and W.W. Franke. 1985a. The complement of desmosomal plaque proteins in different cell types. *J. Cell Biol.* **101:** 1442.

Cowin, P., D. Mattey, and D.R. Garrod. 1984. Identification of desmosomal surface components (desmocollins) and inhibition of desmosome formation by a specific Fab′. *J. Cell Sci.* **70:** 41.

Cowin, P., W.W. Franke, C. Grund, H.-P. Kapprell, and J. Kartenbeck. 1985b. The desmosome-intermediate filament complex. In *The cell in contact* (ed. G. Edelman and J.-P. Thiery), p. 427. Wiley, New York.

Cowin, P., H.-P. Kapprell, W.W. Franke, J. Tamkun, and R.O. Hynes. 1987. Plakoglobin: A protein common to different kinds of intercellular adhering junctions. *Cell* **46**: 1063.

Duden, R. and W.W. Franke. 1988. Organization of desmosomal plaque proteins in cells growing at low calcium concentrations. *J. Cell Biol.* **107**: 1049.

Eyre, R.W. and J.R. Stanley. 1987. Human autoantibodies against a desmosomal protein complex with a calcium-sensitive epitope are characteristic of pemphigus foliaceus patients. *J. Exp. Med.* **165**: 1719.

Farquhar, M.G. and G.E. Palade. 1963. Junctional complexes in various epithelia. *J. Cell Biol.* **17**: 375.

Giudice, G.J., S.M. Cohen, N.H. Patel, and M.S. Steinberg. 1984. Immunological comparison of desmosomal component from several bovine tissues. *J. Cell. Biochem.* **26**: 35.

Gorbsky, G. and M.S. Steinberg. 1981. Isolation of intercellular glycoproteins of desmosomes. *J. Cell Biol.* **90**: 243.

Gorbsky, G., S.M. Cohen, H. Shida, G.J. Giudice, and M.S. Steinberg. 1985. Isolation of the non-glycosylated proteins of the desmosome and immunolocalization of a third plaque protein: Desmoplakin III. *Proc. Natl. Acad. Sci.* **82**: 810.

Green, K.J., R.D. Goldman, and R.L. Chisholm. 1988. Isolation of cDNAs encoding desmosomal plaque proteins: Evidence that bovine desmoplakins I and II are derived from two mRNAs and a single gene. *Proc. Natl. Acad. Sci.* **85**: 2613.

Jones, J.C.R. 1988. Characterization of a 125K glycoprotein associated with bovine epithelial desmosomes. *J. Cell Sci.* **89**: 207.

Jones, J.C.R. and R.D. Goldman. 1985. Intermediate filaments and initiation of desmosome assembly. *J. Cell Biol.* **101**: 506.

Jones, J.C.R., K.M. Yokoo, and R.D. Goldman. 1986. Further analysis of pemphigus autoantibodies and their use in studies on the heterogeneity structure and function of desmosomes. *Proc. Natl. Acad. Sci.* **83**: 7282.

Kapprell, H.-P., K. Owaribe, and W.W. Franke. 1988. Identification of a basic protein of Mr 75,000 as an accessory desmosomal plaque protein in stratified and complex epithelia. *J. Cell Biol.* **106**: 1679.

Kapprell, H.-P., P. Cowin, W.W. Franke, H. Ponstingl, and H.J. Opferkuch. 1985. Biochemical characterization of desmosomal proteins isolated from bovine muzzle epithelium: Amino acid and carbohydrate composition. *Eur. J. Cell Biol.* **36**: 217.

Mattey, D.L. and D.R. Garrod. 1985. Desmosomal formation between all binary combinations of human, bovine, canine, avian, and amphibian cells: Desomosome formation is not tissue- or species-specific. *J. Cell Sci.* **75**: 377.

Miller, K., D. Mattey, M. Measures, C. Hopkins, and D. Garrod. 1987. Localization of the protein and glycoprotein components of bovine nasal epithelial desmosomes by immunoelectron microscopy. *EMBO J.* **6**: 885.

Moll, R., P. Cowin, H.-P. Kapprell, and W.W. Franke. 1986. Desmosomal proteins — New markers for identification and classification
of tumours. *Lab. Invest.* **54:** 4.

Muller, H. and W.W. Franke. 1983. Biochemical and immunological
characterizations of desmoplakins I and II: The major polypeptides
of the desmosomal plaque. *J. Mol. Biol.* **163:** 647.

Parrish, E.P., D.R. Garrod, D.L. Mattey, L. Hand, P.V. Steart, and
R.O. Weller. 1986. Mouse antisera specific for desmosomal adhe-
sion molecules of suprabasal skin cells, meninges and meningioma.
Proc. Natl. Acad. Sci. **83:** 2657.

Pasdar, M. and W.J. Nelson. 1988a. Kinetics of desmosome assembly
in Madin-Derby canine kidney epithelial cells: Temporal and spatial regulation of desmoplakin organisation and stabilization upon
cell-cell contact. I. Biochemical analysis. *J. Cell Biol.* **106:** 677.

————. 1988b. Kinetics of desmosomal assembly in Madin-Derby
canine kidney epithelial cells: Temporal and spatial regulation of
desmoplakin organisation and stabilization upon cell-cell contact.
II. Morphological analysis. *J. Cell. Biol.* **106:** 687.

Penn, E.J., C. Hobson, D.A. Rees, and A.I. Magee. 1987. Structure and
assembly of desmosome junctions: Biosynthesis processing and
transport of the major protein and glycoprotein components in cultured epithelial cells. *J. Cell Biol.* **105:** 57.

Penn, E.J., I.D.J. Burdett, C. Hobson, A.I. Magee, and D.A. Rees.
1988. Structure and assembly of desmosome junctions: Biosynthesis and turnover of the major desmosome components of Madin-
Derby canine kidney cells in low calcium medium. *J. Cell Biol.* **105:**
2327.

Schmelz, M., R. Duden, P. Cowin, and W.W. Franke. 1986a. A constitutive transmembrane glycoprotein of Mr 165,000 (desmoglein) in
epidermal and non-epidermal desmosomes. I. Biochemical identification of the polypeptide. *Eur. J. Cell Biol.* **42:** 177.

————. 1986b. A constitutive transmembrane glycoprotein of Mr
165,000 (desmoglein) in epidermal and non-epidermal desmosomes. II. Immunolocalization and microinjection studies. *Eur. J.
Cell Biol.* **42:** 184.

Steinberg, M.S., M. Shida, G.J. Giudice, M. Shida, N.H. Portel, and
O.W. Blaschuk. 1987. On the molecular organisation, diversity and
functions of desmosomal proteins. *Ciba Found. Symp.* **125:** 3.

Tsukita, S. and S. Tsukita. 1985. Desmocalmin — A calmodulin-
binding high molecular weight protein isolated from desmosomes.
J. Cell Biol. **101:** 2070.

————. 1988. Cell-cell adherens junction. II. Purification and characterization of a new 82kd protein. *Cell Biol. Abstr.* **2:** 18.

Ungar, F., B. Geiger, and A. Ben-Ze'ev. 1986. Cell contact and shape
dependent regulation of vinallin synthesis in cultured fibroblasts.
Nature **319:** 787.

Volk, T., O. Cohen, and B. Geiger. 1987. Formation of heterotypic
adherens-type junctions between L-CAM-containing liver cells and
A-CAM containing lens cells. *Cell* **50:** 987.

Cell-adhesion Molecules

B.A. Cunningham

Laboratory of Developmental and Molecular Biology
The Rockefeller University, New York, New York 10021

Cell adhesion is a primary process in embryonic development and in maintaining the integrity of adult tissues. Over the last decade, cell-surface glycoproteins that mediate these events have been characterized and have provided surprising new insights into the nature and diversity of cell-adhesion molecules (CAMs) and their function (Edelman 1988a). Moreover, CAMs and their genes promise to provide a vast array of new tools for examining other cellular processes and more clinical applications such as tumor detection and diagnosis.

Since the identification of the neural cell-adhesion molecule, N-CAM (Thiery et al. 1977), a number of CAMs (Edelman 1988a) have been found in a wide variety of tissues. Relatively few different molecules have been identified, however, and nearly all of these can be grouped in one of two classes: one resembling N-CAM, and the other resembling the liver cell-adhesion molecule, L-CAM (Gallin et al. 1987). The primary CAMs, N-CAM and L-CAM, are both expressed on the earliest embryonic cells; but as development proceeds, they are differentially seen in distinct cell populations (Crossin et al. 1985). This selective expression is particularly apparent at sites of embryonic induction, where a population of cells expressing one CAM is nearly always found adjacent to a population of cells expressing the other CAM or both CAMs. In adult tissues, N-CAM and L-CAM are detected on different tissues, but both are expressed on cells derived from all three germ layers. In contrast, secondary CAMs, such as the neuron-glia CAM (Ng-CAM) (Grumet and Edelman 1988), are expressed later in development and are much more restricted in their tissue distributions. These findings have suggested (Edelman 1984) that regulation of CAM expression and modulation of CAM activity at specific times are critical in directing and regulating developmental processes.

Although initially found in brain, N-CAM is also expressed transiently in a variety of embryonic tissues and in adult heart, kidney, skeletal muscle, and smooth muscle. The amount and

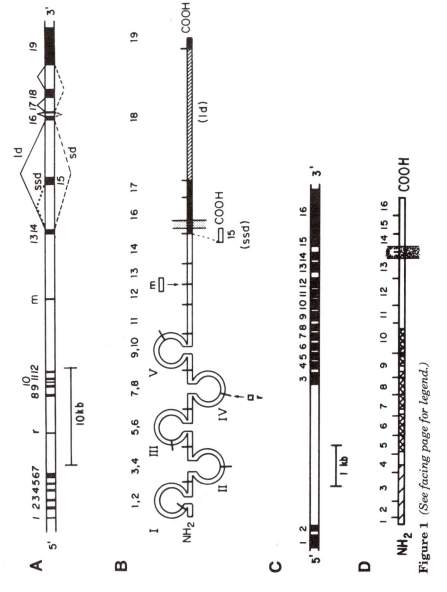

Figure 1 (See facing page for legend.)

192

form of N-CAM expressed are also influenced by cellular transformation (Greenberg et al. 1984) and are altered in certain tumors (Roth et al. 1988). As a glycoprotein, N-CAM is unusual in that it has large amounts of polysialic acid covalently attached to asparagine-linked oligosaccharides (Cunningham et al. 1987). The amount of sialic acid is greatest in N-CAM from embryonic brain (130 moles/mole protein) and decreases as the embryo matures, so that N-CAM in most adult tissues has only about one-third the amount found in embryos (Rothbard et al. 1982). This embryonic (E) to adult (A) conversion occurs in all known forms of N-CAM and is apparently due to a decrease in the activity of one or more sialyl transferases (Friedlander et al. 1985). In different brain regions, the rate of E to A conversion parallels the maturation of each region (Edelman and Chuong 1982), suggesting that it plays an important role in development. In accord with this notion, the conversion leads to enhanced N-CAM binding (Hoffman and Edelman 1983).

Initially, three N-CAM polypeptides were described in chick brain, but other polypeptides are known to exist. All are derived from a single gene, located on chromosome 9 in mice (D'Eustachio et al. 1985) and chromosome 11 in humans (Nguyen et al. 1985). The gene (Fig. 1A) in chickens (Owens et al. 1987) is large (>50 kb), with more than 19 exons utilized in the

Figure 1 Schematic drawings of N-CAM and L-CAM and their genes. (A) The chicken N-CAM gene with exons (black boxes) numbered. All known polypetides utilize exons 1–14. The exons that are differentially spliced to give the ld polypeptide (solid lines), the sd polypeptide (broken line), and the ssd polypeptide (dotted line) are indicated as are the positions where exons for inserts seen in N-CAM from human muscle (m) and rat brain (r) would be located in the chicken gene. (B) Composite of structural elements of N-CAM polypeptides, with segments unique to the ld and ssd polypeptides and the locations of inserts seen in human muscle (m) and rat brain polypeptides (r) indicated. The ssd polypeptide is attached to the membrane (stippled vertical bar) by a phospholipid anchor, whereas the ld and sd polypeptides are integral membrane proteins. The loops (I–V) denote immunoglobulin-like regions, and the lines denote the boundaries of exons (numbered above). (C) The L-CAM gene with exons (black boxes) numbered; note the difference in scale with A. (D) L-CAM polypeptide, with the sequence unique to the precursor (hatching) and homologous segments (crosshatching) indicated. Vertical lines denote boundaries of exons (numbered above); the membrane (stippled vertical bar)-spanning segment includes the boundary between exons 13 and 14.

coding regions (Fig. 1B). The smallest N-CAM polypeptide, small surface domain (ssd) polypeptide, is specified by exons 1–15; it is attached to cell membranes by a phosphatidylinositol lipid anchor (Hemperly et al. 1986a; He et al. 1986) and appears to be synthesized primarily in glial cells. The next larger polypeptide, small cytoplasmic domain (sd) polypeptide (Cunningham et al. 1987), is specified by exons 1–14 plus exons 16, 17, and 19, whereas the large cytoplasmic domain (ld) polypeptide includes an additional cytoplasmic sequence specified by exon 18. Both of these larger chains are integral membrane proteins that are phosphorylated on serine and threonine residues and can incorporate fatty acids (Sorkin et al. 1984). The largest polypeptide (ld) is expressed preferentially in neurons (Pollerberg et al. 1985; Murray et al. 1986) and interacts selectively with brain spectrin (Pollerberg et al. 1986). N-CAM polypeptides from other animal species (Barthels et al. 1987; Dickson et al. 1987; Santoni et al. 1987; Small et al. 1987) are all closely related to each other and to the chicken N-CAM polypeptides (>80% amino acid identity), consistent with earlier observations (Hoffman et al. 1984) that N-CAMs from different species bind to each other. Studies in other species have also revealed additional forms of N-CAM, including an ssd-like polypeptide in human muscle (Dickson et al. 1987) that has a 37-amino-acid insert at a position equivalent to the junction of exons 12 and 13 (Fig. 1B), and an sd-like chain in rat brain (Small et al. 1987) that has a 10-amino-acid insert at a position equivalent to the junction of exons 7 and 8.

The extracellular regions of all known N-CAM polypeptides (Cunningham et al. 1987) contain five contiguous segments (Fig. 1B) that resemble immunoglobulin (Ig) domains (Williams 1987; Edelman 1988b). This portion of N-CAM includes the binding region, and N-CAM binding probably involves the interaction of two or more of the first four (I–IV) Ig-like domains; the sites for attachment of the polysialic acid are in domain V. From domain V to the cell membrane, the amino acid sequence resembles type III repeats in fibronectin (Petersen et al. 1983; Hemperly et al. 1986b). The relationship of N-CAM to Igs has important implications for understanding the evolution of the Ig supergene family (Edelman 1988b) and establishes a basis for a family of related CAMs. The myelin-associated glycoprotein (MAG) (Arquint et al. 1987; Lai et al. 1987; Salzer et al. 1987), the myelin-associated protein, P_0 (Lemke and Axel 1985), the neural glycoprotein L-1 (Moos et al. 1988), and the

ICAM-1 (Simmons et al. 1988) molecule all have structures similar to that of N-CAM and all have putative cell-adhesion functions. Therefore, it appears that there is a family of primary and secondary CAMs whose binding functions depend on the interactions of Ig-like domains.

L-CAM is an integral membrane protein (Gallin et al. 1987) that appears on nearly all epithelia, although it is only rarely seen in neural epithelia (Levi et al. 1987). In contrast to N-CAM, L-CAM has been detected in only one molecular form in all tissues in which it is expressed (Thiery et al. 1984; Gallin et al. 1987); it contains no polysialic acid and appears to be the product of a single, much smaller (10 kb) gene (Sorkin et al. 1988). The structural gene (Fig. 1C) in chickens contains 16 exons, but there is no evidence for alternative splicing and the exon boundaries do not correspond to known structural features of the protein (Fig. 1D). L-CAM is initially synthesized as a larger precursor (M_r = 135,000) that is rapidly trimmed at the amino-terminal end with concomitant changes in carbohydrate and phosphorylation to yield the M_r 124,000 form that is expressed on the cell surface. L-CAM contains no Ig-like segments, but it includes three contiguous segments of about 110 amino acids that are 20–40% identical to each other, suggesting that the evolution of the molecule involved one or more duplication events (Gallin et al. 1987). Calcium is important both to the L-CAM structure and to its binding, and the molecule binds calcium (Ringwald et al. 1987). Proteins with similar activities, tissue distributions, and chemical properties have been identified in humans (Damsky et al. 1983), mice (Hyafil et al. 1981; Yoshida and Takeichi 1982), and dogs (Imhof et al. 1983), and they are assumed to be homologs of chicken L-CAM; the amino acid sequence of the protein from mouse has been determined (Nagafuchi et al. 1987; Ringwald et al. 1987) and closely resembles (70% identical) that of chicken L-CAM.

L-CAM (and its homologs) is the first of a family of closely related proteins that mediates calcium-dependent adhesion. Other members of this family include N-cadherin (Shirayoshi et al. 1986) and adherens (A)-CAM (Volk and Geiger 1986), found in chicken brain, lens, and heart. Another such molecule is P-cadherin (Nose et al. 1987), which was detected initially in a mouse visceral endoderm cell line and is prominent on placenta. These molecules differ from L-CAM and each other in their tissue distributions and binding specificities (Hirano et al. 1987), and they are synthesized from different genes; but they are very similar (50% identity) to L-CAM and to each other in amino acid sequence (Shirayoshi et al. 1986; Nose et al. 1987).

Earlier studies suggested that the binding mechanisms of both N-CAM and L-CAM are homophilic, i.e., a CAM on one cell binds the same CAM on apposing cells. This conclusion has now been strengthened by expressing N-CAM or L-CAM cDNAs in cell lines that do not normally express them (Edelman et al. 1987; Hirano et al. 1987). Mouse L cells transfected with plasmids containing the SV40 early promoter and cDNAs encoding chicken L-CAM or N-CAM expressed the appropriate proteins at the cell surfaces. Transfected cells aggregated to cells expressing the same CAM, but not to cells expressing the other CAM or to untransfected L cells, and aggregation was inhibited by the appropriate antibodies. Cellular transfection has also provided further evidence that CAM expression influences phenotypic alterations at several levels. For example (Mege et al. 1988), when mouse S180 sarcoma cells were transfected with a vector encoding chicken L-CAM, the cells were changed to a polygonal shape and formed tightly linked epithelioid sheets, with L-CAM concentrated at sites of cell-cell contact and colocalized with cortical actin. Ultrastructural and dye-coupling studies showed a marked increase in the number of adherens junctions and the number and size of functional gap junctions. These results imply a close link between CAM function and other fundamental cellular processes — a link that is most likely mediated by cytoplasmic components, including elements of the cytoskeleton.

REFERENCES

Arquint, M., S. Roder, L.S. Chia, J. Down, D. Wilkinson, H. Bayley, P. Braun, and R. Dunn. 1987. Molecular cloning and primary structure of myelin-associated glycoprotein. *Proc. Natl. Acad. Sci.* **84:** 600.

Barthels, D., M.-J. Santoni, W. Wille, C. Ruppert, J.-C. Chaix, R. Hirsch, J.C. Fontecilla-Camps, and C. Goridis. 1987. Isolation and nucleotide sequence of mouse NCAM cDNA that codes for a Mr 79,000 polypeptide without a membrane-spanning region. *EMBO J.* **6:** 907.

Crossin, K.L., C.-M. Chuong, and G.M. Edelman. 1985. Expression sequences of cell adhesion molecules. *Proc. Natl. Acad. Sci.* **82:** 6942.

Cunningham, B.A., J.J. Hemperly, B.A. Murray, E.A. Prediger, R. Brackenbury, and G.M. Edelman. 1987. Neural cell adhesion molecule: Structure, immunoglobulin-like domains, cell surface modulation, and alternative RNA splicing. *Science* **236:** 799.

Damsky, C.H., J. Richa, D. Solter, K. Knudsen, and C.A. Buck. 1983.

Identification and purification of a cell surface glycoprotein involved in cell-cell interactions. *Cell* **34**: 455.

D'Eustachio, P., G. Owens, G.M. Edelman, and B.A. Cunningham. 1985. Chromosomal location of the gene encoding the neural cell adhesion molecule N-CAM in the mouse. *Proc. Natl. Acad. Sci.* **82**: 7631.

Dickson, G., H.J. Gower, C.H. Barton, H.M. Prentice, V.L. Elsom, S.E. Moore, R.D. Cox, C. Quinn, W. Putt, and F. Walsh. 1987. Human muscle neural cell adhesion molecule N-CAM: Identification of a muscle specific sequence in the extracellular domain. *Cell* **50**: 1119.

Edelman, G.M. 1984. Cell adhesion and morphogenesis: The regulator hypothesis. *Proc. Natl. Acad. Sci.* **81**: 1460.

———. 1988a. Morphoregulatory molecules. *Biochemistry* **27**: 3533.

———. 1988b. CAMs and Igs: Cell adhesion and the evolutionary origins of immunity. *Immunol. Rev.* **100**: 11.

Edelman, G.M. and C.-M. Chuong. 1982. Embryonic to adult conversion of neural cell-adhesion molecules in normal and *staggerer* mice. *Proc. Natl. Acad. Sci.* **79**: 7036.

Edelman, G.M., B.A. Murray, R.-M. Mege, B.A. Cunningham, and W.J. Gallin. 1987. Cellular expression of liver and neural cell adhesion molecules after transfection with their cDNAs results in specific cell-cell binding. *Proc. Natl. Acad. Sci.* **84**: 8502.

Friedlander, D.R., R. Brackenbury, and G.M. Edelman. 1985. Conversion of embryonic forms of N-CAM *in vitro* results from *de novo* synthesis of adult forms. *J. Cell Biol.* **101**: 412.

Gallin, W.J., B.C. Sorkin, G.M. Edelman, and B.A. Cunningham. 1987. Sequence analysis of a cDNA clone encoding the liver cell adhesion molecule, L-CAM. *Proc. Natl. Acad. Sci.* **84**: 2808.

Greenberg, M.E., R. Brackenbury, and G.M. Edelman. 1984. Alteration of neural cell adhesion molecules (N-CAM) expression after neuronal cell transformation by Rous sarcoma virus. *Proc. Natl. Acad. Sci.* **81**: 969.

Grumet, M. and G.M. Edelman. 1988. Neuron-glia cell adhesion molecule interacts with neurons and astroglia via different binding mechanisms. *J. Cell Biol.* **106**: 487.

He, H.T., J. Barbet, J.C. Chaix, and C. Goridis. 1986. Phosphatidylinositol is involved in the membrane attachment of NCAM-120, the smallest component of the neural cell adhesion molecule. *EMBO J.* **5**: 2489.

Hemperly, J.J., G.M. Edelman, and B.A. Cunningham. 1986a. cDNA clones of the neural cell adhesion molecule (N-CAM) lacking a membrane-spanning region consistent with evidence for membrane attachment via a phosphatidylinositol intermediate. *Proc. Natl. Acad. Sci.* **83**: 9822.

Hemperly, J.J., B.A. Murray, G.M. Edelman, and B.A. Cunningham. 1986b. Sequence of a cDNA clone encoding the polysialic acid-rich and cytoplasmic domains of the neural cell adhesion molecule N-CAM. *Proc. Natl. Acad. Sci.* **83**: 3037.

Hirano, S., A. Nose, K. Hatta, A. Kawakami, and M. Takeichi. 1987. Calcium-dependent cell-cell adhesion molecules (cadherins): Subclass specificities and possible involvement of actin bundles. *J. Cell Biol.* **105**: 2501.

Hoffman, S. and G.M. Edelman. 1983. Kinetics of homophilic binding by E and A forms of the neural cell adhesion molecule. *Proc. Natl. Acad. Sci.* **80:** 5762.

Hoffman, S., C.-M. Chuong, and G.M. Edelman. 1984. Evolutionary conservation of key structures and binding functions of neural cell adhesion molecules. *Proc. Natl. Acad. Sci.* **81:** 6881.

Hyafil, F., C. Babinet, and F. Jacob. 1981. Cell-cell interactions in early embryogenesis: A molecular approach to the role of calcium. *Cell* **26:** 447.

Imhof, B.A., H.P. Vollmers, S.L. Goodman, and W. Birchmeier. 1983. Cell-cell interaction and polarity of epithelial cells: Specific perturbation using a monoclonal antibody. *Cell* **35:** 667.

Lai, C., M.A. Brow, K.-A. Nave, A.B. Noronha, R.H. Quarles, F.E. Bloom, R.J. Milner, and J.G. Sutcliffe. 1987. Two forms of 1B236/myelin-associated glycoprotein, a cell adhesion molecule for postnatal neural development, are produced by alternative splicing. *Proc. Natl. Acad. Sci.* **84:** 4337.

Lemke, G. and R. Axel. 1985. Isolation and sequence of a cDNA encoding the major structural protein of peripheral myelin. *Cell* **40:** 501.

Levi, G., K.L. Crossin, and G.M. Edelman. 1987. Expression sequences and distribution of two primary cell adhesion molecules during embryonic development of *Xenopus laevis*. *J. Cell Biol.* **105:** 2359.

Mege, R.-M., F. Matsuzaki, W.J. Gallin, J.I. Goldberg, B.A. Cunningham, and G.M. Edelman. 1988. Construction of epithelioid sheets by transfection of mouse sarcoma cells with cDNAs for chicken cell adhesion molecules. *Proc. Natl. Acad. Sci.* **85:** 7274.

Moos, M., R. Tacke, H. Scherer, D. Teplow, K. Früh, and M. Schachner. 1988. Neural adhesion molecule L1 as a member of the immunoglobulin superfamily with binding domains similar to fibronectin. *Nature* **334:** 701.

Murray, B.A., G.C. Owens, E.A. Prediger, K.L. Crossin, B.A. Cunningham, and G.M. Edelman. 1986. Cell surface modulation of the neuronal cell adhesion molecule resulting from alternative mRNA splicing in a tissue-specific developmental sequence. *J. Cell Biol.* **103:** 1431.

Nagafuchi, A., Y. Shirayoshi, K. Okazaki, K. Yasuda, and M. Takeichi. 1987. Transformation of cell adhesion properties by exogenously introduced E-cadherin cDNA. *Nature* **329:** 341.

Nguyen, C., M.G. Mattei, C. Goridis, J.F. Mattei, and B.R. Jordan. 1985. Localization of the human N-CAM gene to chromosome 11 by *in situ* hybridization with a murine N-CAM cDNA probe. *Cytogenet. Cell Genet.* **40:** 713.

Nose, A., A. Nagafuchi, and M. Takeichi. 1987. Isolation of placental cadherin cDNA: Identification of a novel gene family of cell-cell adhesion molecules. *EMBO J.* **6:** 3655.

Owens, G.C., G.M. Edelman, and B.A. Cunningham. 1987. Organization of the neural cell adhesion molecule N-CAM gene: Alternative exon usage as the basis for different membrane-associated domains. *Proc. Natl. Acad. Sci.* **84:** 294.

Petersen, T.E., H.C. Thøgersen, K. Skorstengaard, K. Vibe-Pedersen, P. Sahl, L. Sottrup-Jensen, and S. Magnusson. 1983. Partial primary structure of bovine plasma fibronectin, three types of internal homology. *Proc. Natl. Acad. Sci.* **80:** 137.

Pollerberg, E.G., M. Schachner, and S. Davoust. 1986. Differentiation state-dependent surface mobilities of two forms of the neural cell adhesion molecule. *Nature* **324:** 462.

Pollerberg, E.G., R. Sadoul, C. Goridis, and M. Schachner. 1985. Selective expression of the 180-KD component of the neural cell-adhesion molecule N-CAM during development. *J. Cell Biol.* **101:** 1921.

Ringwald, M., R. Schuh, D. Vestweber, H. Eistetter, F. Lottspeich, J. Engel, R. Dölz, F. Jähnig, J. Eppler, S. Mayer, C. Müller, and R. Kemler. 1987. The structure of cell adhesion molecule uvomorulin. Insights into the molecular mechanism of CA^{2+}-dependent cell adhesion. *EMBO J.* **6:** 3647.

Roth, J., C. Zuber, P. Wagner, D.J. Taatjes, C. Weisberger, P.U. Heitz, C. Goridis, and D. Bitter-Suerman. 1988. Reexpression of poly(sialic acid) units of the neural cell adhesion molecule in Wilms tumor. *Proc. Natl. Acad. Sci.* **85:** 2999.

Rothbard, J.B., R. Brackenbury, B.A. Cunningham, and G.M. Edelman. 1982. Differences in the carbohydrate structures of neural cell adhesion molecules from adult and embryonic chicken brains. *J. Biol. Chem.* **257:** 11064.

Salzer, J.G., W.P. Holmes, and D.R. Colman. 1987. The amino acid sequences of the myelin-associated glycoproteins: Homology to the immunoglobulin gene superfamily. *J. Cell Biol.* **104:** 957.

Santoni, M.-J., D. Barthels, J.A. Barbas, M.-R. Hirsh, M. Steinmetz, C. Goridis, and W. Wille. 1987. Analysis of cDNA clones that code for the transmembrane forms of the mouse neural cell adhesion molecule (NCAM) and are generated by alternative RNA splicing. *Nucleic Acids Res.* **15:** 8621.

Shirayoshi, Y., K. Hatta, M. Hosoda, S. Tsunasawa, F. Sakiyama, and M. Takeichi. 1986. Cadherin cell adhesion molecules with distinct binding specificities share a common structure. *EMBO J.* **5:** 2485.

Simmons, D., M.W. Makgoba, and B. Seed. 1988. ICAM, an adhesion ligand of LFA-1, is homologous to NCAM. *Nature* **331:** 624.

Small, S.J., G.E. Shull, M.-J. Santoni, and R. Akeson. 1987. Identification of a cDNA clone that contains the complete coding sequence for a 140-kD rat NCAM polypeptide. *J. Cell Biol.* **105:** 2335.

Sorkin, B.C., J.J. Hemperly, G.M. Edelman, and B.A. Cunningham. 1988. Structure of the gene for the liver cell adhesion molecule, L-CAM. *Proc. Natl. Acad. Sci.* **85:** 7617.

Sorkin, B.C., S. Hoffman, G.M. Edelman, and B.A. Cunningham. 1984. Sulfation and phosphorylation of the neural cell adhesion molecule N-CAM. *Science* **225:** 1476.

Thiery, J.-P., R. Brackenbury, U. Rutishauser, and G.M. Edelman. 1977. Adhesion among neural cells of the chick embryo. II. Purification and characterization of a cell adhesion molecule from neural retina. *J. Biol. Chem.* **252:** 6841.

Thiery, J.-P., A. Delouvée, W.J. Gallin, B.A. Cunningham, and G.M. Edelman. 1984. Ontogenetic expression of cell adhesion molecules: L-CAM is found in epithelia derived from the three primary germ layers. *Dev. Biol.* **102:** 61.

Volk, T. and B. Geiger. 1986. A-CAM: A 136 kd receptor of intercellular adherens junctions. I. Immuno-electron microscopic localization and biochemical studies. *J. Cell Biol.* **103:** 1441.

Williams, A.F. 1987. A year in the life of the immunoglobulin superfamily. *Immunol. Today* **8:** 298.

Yoshida, C. and M. Takeichi. 1982. Teratocarcinoma cell adhesion: Identification of a cell-surface protein involved in calcium-dependent cell aggregation. *Cell* **28:** 217.

Use of Villin for the Histopathological and Serological Diagnosis of Digestive Cancers

D. Louvard, M. Arpin, E. Coudrier,
B. Dudouet, J. Finidori, A. Garcia,
C. Huet, R. Maunoury, E. Pringault,
S. Robine, and C. Sahuquillo-Merino

Département de Biologie Moléculaire, Unité de Biologie
des Membranes, Institut Pasteur, 75724 Paris Cedex 15, France

Over the last decade, studies devoted to the cellular and molecular biology of structural proteins associated with intermediate filaments, as well as findings on several proteins involved in the cytoplasmic organization of cells, have convincingly established the value of these cellular components for tumor classification (see data reported in this volume).

Cell biologists and pathologists have a pressing need for well-characterized monoclonal antibodies against well-defined antigens. These molecular probes can be useful, for example, to establish the origin of cells. In cell biology, these antibodies can be used for the analysis of cell lineages during embryogenesis or to identify cells in culture. In pathology, these reagents provide a useful adjunct for the identification and classification of tumors.

Our research on the cellular and molecular biology of digestive epithelial cells led us to study the properties of villin, a structural component of enterocytes. Several observations made in our laboratory suggested further investigation of the usefulness of villin as a marker for the histopathological and serological diagnosis of digestive cancers.

Here, we report some properties of villin and results supporting our original proposal that villin is a differentiation marker of epithelial intestinal cells that also has some value in studies on human digestive cancers (Robine et al. 1985).

Villin Is a Calcium-regulated Actin-binding Protein

Villin was first described by A. Bretscher in Klaus Weber's laboratory in 1979; it is a monomeric, globular nonglycosylated

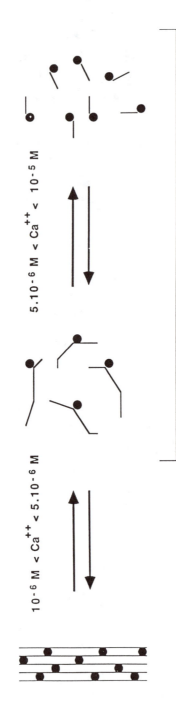

" BUNDLING"

10^{-6} M < Ca^{++} < 5.10^{-6} M

5.10^{-6} M < Ca^{++} < 10^{-5} M

" SEVERING"

Figure 1 In vitro interaction of villin with F-actin.

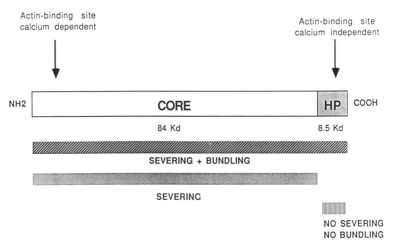

Figure 2 Functional domains of chicken villin.

protein (92.5 kD) (Bretscher and Weber 1980; Craig and Powell 1980; Mooseker et al. 1980). In vitro, villin binds to F actin in a calcium-dependent manner. When the calcium concentration is below 10^{-6} to 10^{-7} M, villin acts as a bundling factor. At micromolar concentration, villin leads to the formation of short F-actin microfilaments by preventing monomer addition and forming at the barbed end what is known as a functional cap. Villin severs actin microfilaments at concentrations above 10 μM (Fig. 1). Different actin-binding sites have been mapped on the protein using protease treatments. Using the V8 protease, Glenney et al. (1981) cleaved chicken villin into two fragments with apparent molecular masses of 90 and 8.5 kD. The largest fragment, called the villin core, has a Ca^{++}-dependent nucleation and severing actin-binding activities but does not bundle actin filaments (Fig. 2). The smallest fragment, called the "head piece," is located at the carboxyl terminus of villin; it binds to actin regardless of the presence of calcium in the medium and has no bundling or severing activities (Fig. 2).

Full-length cDNAs coding for chicken and human villin have been isolated, allowing determination of the complete amino acid sequences (Arpin et al. 1988; Bazari et al. 1988). Chicken and human villin display 80% homology in their primary sequences, accounting for the good immunological cross-reactivity between species reported previously (Dudouet et al.

203

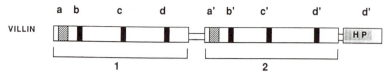

Figure 3 Schematic representation of the structural organization of human villin.

1987; Fiegel et al. 1987). The analysis of the villin sequence shows the existence of three domains: two large duplicated domains and a small domain corresponding to the head piece (HP; Fig. 3). Each duplicated domain displays four internal motifs; three of them present similarities with each other. These motifs are regularly separated from each other by a stretch of about 100 amino acids along the molecule (Fig. 3, bb', cc', dd', solid bar). The fourth motif is found near the amino terminus of each large domain and has no internal homology with the other repeats (Fig. 3, a, a', hatched bar).

Villin Distribution in Adult Tissues

In contrast to other cytoskeletal proteins found in intestinal brush borders, villin displays striking tissue specificity. The tissue-specific expression of proteins associated with intermediate filaments is well documented. However, such a property has only recently emerged for a few actin-binding proteins and their isoforms (see Gabbiani; Morrow et al.; both this volume). Using antibodies raised against villin, we have shown by immunocytochemical and immunochemical procedures that the occurrence of this protein is restricted to a few epithelial cells of urogenital and gastrointestinal tracts (Robine et al. 1985; Moll et al. 1987). It was first demonstrated that cells having a brush border contain a large amount of this protein accumulated at their apex (Bretscher and Weber 1979; Reggio et al. 1982). By ultrastructural immunolabeling, we have shown that villin is localized along the entire length of the microvilli microfilament bundles in differentiated intestinal cells (Dudouet et al. 1987). However, biliary and pancreatic duct cells lacking an organized brush border express low levels of villin, localized beneath their apical borders (Robine et al. 1985). These findings prompted us to investigate the time and the location of villin appearance during embryogenesis to establish a possible relationship between villin expression and cellular morphogenesis.

Villin Expression during Mouse Embryogenesis

During the course of mouse embryonic development, villin expression is precisely modulated. The regulation of villin expression concerns the time and cell types that are able to produce villin. Briefly, villin first appears in the visceral endoderm at day 5–6 of mouse embryogenesis. The visceral endoderm (also called proximal endoderm or yolk sac) is a polarized differentiated simple epithelium surrounding the embryo proper. This epithelium achieves the functions of a primitive intestine because it transports nutrients produced by the mother to the developing embryo (Maunoury et al. 1988). As soon as the intestinal tube appears, the endodermic cells constituting the primitive intestine express villin. In this multilayer of undifferentiated cells, villin is expressed and uniformly distributed throughout the cytoplasm. Production of villin is strikingly increased when terminal differentiation of intestinal cells is set up in late embryogenesis. Simultaneously, during this process, villin is recruited at the apical borders of differentiating cells. This sequence of events is reminiscent of our observations on villin expression along the crypt villus axis in the adult intestine or in differentiating intestinal cells in culture (Robine et al. 1985; Dudouet et al. 1987; Böller et al. 1989). During late embryogenesis, from day 12 until birth, the villin gene is turned on and off in epithelial digestive cells. Primordial cells forming the liver and the pancreatic anlage all express villin, but differentiating embryonic hepatocytes and exocrine or endocrine embryonic acinar pancreatic cells shut off villin production. In contrast, biliary duct cells and pancreatic duct cells continue to produce villin. This profile of villin expression emphasizes the early and controlled expression of villin during development (R. Maunoury et al., unpubl.). These data are schematically summarized in Figure 4.

Here, we have not discussed the expression of villin in primitive and developing kidney proximal tubules, which is the only other location in the embryo and in the adult organism where villin is expressed.

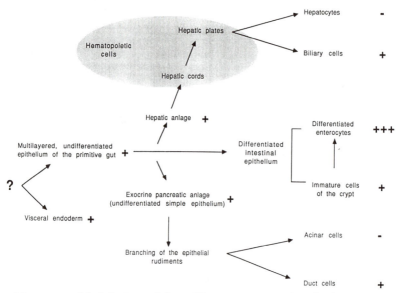

Figure 4 Modulation of the villin gene expression during organogenesis of the digestive tract.

Villin Expression in Malignant Cells

The specificity of villin expression in adult and embryo suggested that we investigate the occurrence of villin in tissue-cultured cells. We have reported that villin was found only in cell lines of intestinal or renal origin, providing that kidney cells in culture displayed some properties of proximal tubular cells (Robine et al. 1985). These observations were further confirmed by Chantret et al. (1988), who showed that the level of villin expression correlated positively with the stage of differentiation of numerous established cell lines derived from human colorectal adenocarcinoma. Moreover, previous studies carried out by others and by us demonstrated that villin is not reexpressed in a wide variety of established cell lines (Bretscher et al. 1981; Robine et al. 1985).

We hypothesized that the cellular specificity of villin reported above may also be observed in human primary tumors. Thus, we assumed that if a specific expression of villin could be demonstrated in human primary tumors, immunocytochemical procedures performed with antibodies against villin could be applied to the classification of tumors derived from tissues that normally express villin. We tested this proposal in collaboration with R. Moll. A large panel of human adenocarcinoma was analyzed for villin expression (Moll et al. 1987). All colorectal adenocarcinoma (primary tumors or metastasis) tested expressed villin, regardless of their stage of differentiation. Similarly, most digestive tumors produced from cells that usually express villin were positively detected (pancreatic adenocarcinoma, cholangioma, and some stomach adenocarcinoma. Accordingly, renal tumors derived from proximal tubular cells were usually found positive. Similar results have been reported by West et al. (1988) and Gröne et al. (1986) for colorectal adenocarcinoma and renal adenocarcinoma, respectively. However, we have noticed two exceptions that cannot be interpreted easily, taking into account our current observations on villin expression in adult and embryonic tissues. Some human endometrium and lung adenocarcinoma were found positive, whereas the corresponding adult or embryonic mouse tissues did not express detectable amounts of villin. We cannot exclude differences between species or an abnormal reexpression of villin in these tumors. Further investigation will be necessary to address these questions. These data are summarized in Figure 5.

Presence of Villin in Human Sera

The tissue-specific expression of villin in adult tissue, as well as its distribution in human primary tumors, led us to investigate its occurrence in human sera. We proposed that cell lysis in necrotic and highly vascularized adenocarcinoma expressing villin might result in release of villin in the bloodstream. To test this hypothesis, almost 800 samples of blood sera were obtained from healthy donors and patients. An ELISA was designed to detect 0.5 ng of villin in human sera. This assay takes advantage of a monoclonal antibody against villin obtained and characterized in our laboratory (Dudouet et al. 1987). The results are summarized in Table 1. Our data show that villin is detected infrequently in the sera of healthy donors, in the sera of patients bearing nondigestive malignant tumors, and in the sera of healthy patients with inflammatory or ulcerative diseases of the gastrointestinal tract. In contrast, up to 50% of patients bearing digestive tumors have abnormal serum villin levels (from 20 to 3000 ng/ml). This applies to patients bearing noninvasive digestive tumors (B stage of

Colon, Rectum	Adenocarcinoma	24*	100%
Stomach	Tubular adenocarc.	6	100%
	Signet-ring-cell/ undifferentiated carc.	3	33% 66%
Pancreas	Adenocarcinoma (duct-cell-type)	14	43% 43%
Gall bladder	Adenocarcinoma	2	
	Adenosquamous carc.	1	
Liver	Hepatocell. carc.	1	
	Cholangiocell. carc.	1	
Kidney	Renal cell carc.		
	Clear cell type, gr.I	4	75% 25%
	Clear cell type, gr II	5	20% 80%
	Clear cell type, grIII	4	25% 75%
	Basoph.cell type (grI,II)	3	
	Eosinoph.cell type (grII)	1	
	Chromoph.cell type (grII)	4	

208

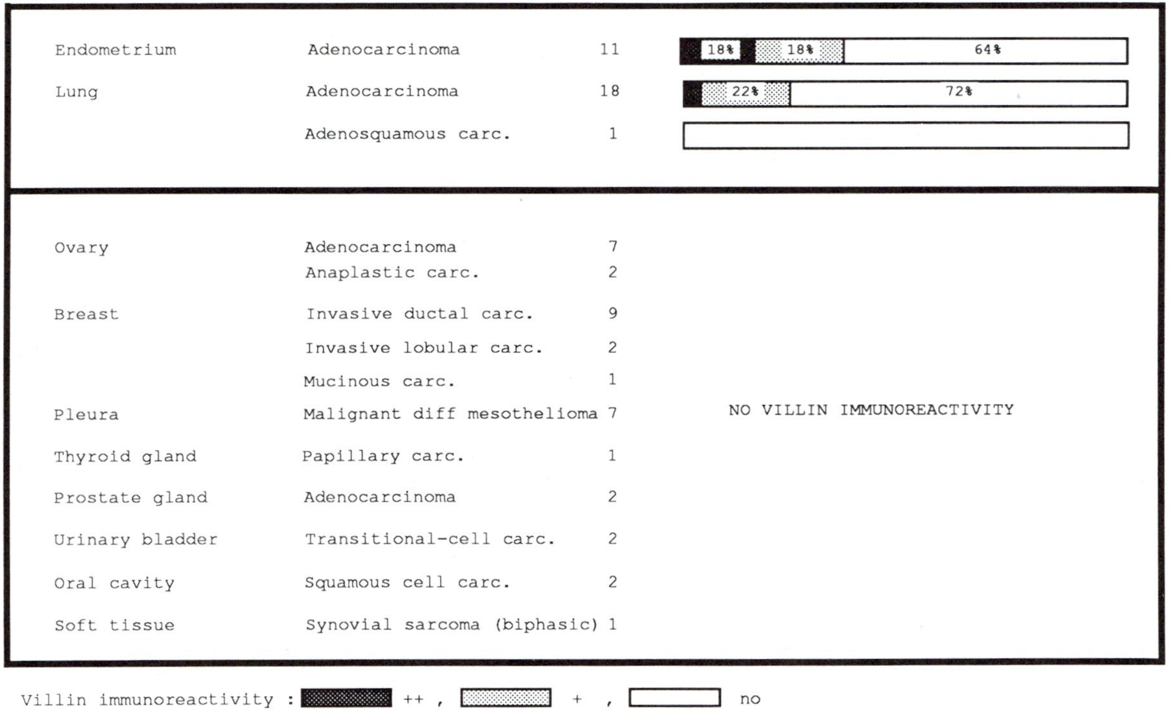

Endometrium	Adenocarcinoma	11	18%	18%	64%
Lung	Adenocarcinoma	18	22%		72%
	Adenosquamous carc.	1			
Ovary	Adenocarcinoma	7			
	Anaplastic carc.	2			
Breast	Invasive ductal carc.	9			
	Invasive lobular carc.	2	NO VILLIN IMMUNOREACTIVITY		
	Mucinous carc.	1			
Pleura	Malignant diff mesothelioma	7			
Thyroid gland	Papillary carc.	1			
Prostate gland	Adenocarcinoma	2			
Urinary bladder	Transitional-cell carc.	2			
Oral cavity	Squamous cell carc.	2			
Soft tissue	Synovial sarcoma (biphasic)	1			

Villin immunoreactivity : ■ ++ , ▨ + , ▢ no

Figure 5 Villin expression in human primary tumors and metastasis. (*) Number of samples tested.

Table 1 Statistical Significance of Villin Detection in Healthy Donors and in Donors with Benign Digestive, Malignant Digestive, and Extradigestive Diseases

Comparison of clinical variables	No. of patients' sera with villin levels above threshold (1)	%	No. of patients' sera with villin levels above threshold (2)	%	χ^2	P
Healthy donors (1) and those with benign digestive diseases (2)	13	3 (13/421)	17	12.8 (17/132)	16.91	<0.001
Healthy donors (1) and those with malignant digestive diseases (2)	13	3 (13/421)	48	50.5 (48/95)	162.81	<<0.001
Donors with benign digestive diseases (1) and malignant digestive diseases (2)	17	12.8 (17/132)	48	50.5 (48/95)	36.49	<0.001
Donors with malignant extra-digestive diseases (1) and malignant digestive diseases (2)	4	5 (4/80)	48	50.5 (48/95)	40.94	<0.001
Healthy donors (1) and those with malignant extra-digestive diseases (2)	13	3 (13/421)	4	5 (4/80)	0.280	NS

Duke's classification). As indicated in Table 1, this value is statistically significant, allowing us to determine a specificity of 94% for the villin assay and a sensitivity of 50% for the panel of sera investigated. Therefore, we concluded that the occurrence of villin in human sera very often is indicative of a pathological state in the gastrointestinal tract.

CONCLUSIONS

Studies carried out on the cellular and molecular biology of villin showed that this actin-binding protein is an early marker of intestinal differentiation. Its tissue-specific expression in several cell lineages allows the use of antibodies against villin as probes for basic studies in cellular biology and development. Moreover, the data reported here suggest that villin is a new marker for studies on digestive cancers. Further work in progress in our laboratory is aimed at analyzing the function of villin in cells able to express it. The availability of antibodies and nucleic acid probes should allow us to dissect further the regulation and disregulation of the expression of this structural protein during embryogenesis, terminal differentiation, and neoplasic transformation of digestive epithelial cells.

ACKNOWLEDGMENTS

We thank Drs. L. Jacob, P. Beuzeboc, H. Magdalenat, Y. Chapuis, B. Christoforov, G. Cremer, P. Pouillard, P. Bonnichon, F. Pinon, R. Salmon, A. Pointereau-Bellanger, and J. Bellanger for their fruitful collaboration in the studies of human sera, and R. Carré for typing this manuscript. This work was supported by grants from the Institut National de la Santé et de la Recherche Médicale (N86-7008), by the Fondation pour la Recherche Médicale Française, by the Association pour la Recherche sur le Cancer (N6379), the Centre Nationale de la Recherche Scientifique (UA-1149), and the Ligue Nationale Française Contre le Cancer.

REFERENCES

Arpin, M., E. Pringault, J. Finidori, A. Garcia, J.M. Jeltsch, V. Vanderkerckhove, and D. Louvard. 1988. Complete sequence of human villin: A large duplicated domain homologous with other actin severing proteins and a unique small carboxy-terminal domain related to villin specificity. *J. Cell Biol.* **107:** 1759.

Bazari, W., P. Matsudaira, M. Wallek, T. Smeal, R. Jakes, and Y.

Ahmed. 1988. Villin sequence and peptide map identify six homologous domains. *Proc. Natl. Acad. Sci.* **85:** 4986.

Böller, K., M. Arpin, E. Pringault, P. Mangeat, and H. Reggio. 1989. Differential distribution of villin and villin m-RNA in mouse intestinal epithelial cells. *Differentiation* (in press).

Bretscher, A. and K. Weber. 1979. Villin: The major microfilament-associated protein of the intestinal microvillus. *Proc. Natl. Acad. Sci.* **76:** 2321.

———. 1980. Villin is a major protein of the microvillus cytoskeleton which binds both G and F actin in a calcium-dependent manner. *Cell* **20:** 839.

Bretscher, A., M. Osborn, J. Wehland, and K. Weber. 1981. Villin associates with specific microfilamentous structures as seen by immunofluorescence microscopy on tissue sections and cells microinjected with villin. *Exp. Cell Res.* **135:** 213.

Chantret, I., A. Barbat, E. Dussaulx, M.G. Brattain, and A. Zweibaum. 1988. Epithelial polarity, villin expression and enterocytic differentiation of cultured human colon carcinoma cells: A survey of 20 cell lines. *Cancer Res.* **48:** 1936.

Craig, S.W. and L.D. Powell. 1980. Comparison of intestinal brush-border 95-kDalton polypeptide and alpha-actinins. *Cell* **22:** 739.

Dudouet, B., S. Robine, C. Huet, C. Sahuquillo-Merino, L. Blair, E. Coudrier, and D. Louvard. 1987. Changes in villin synthesis and subcellular distribution during intestinal differentiation of HT29-18 clones. *J. Cell Biol.* **105:** 359.

Fiegel, A., J. Schilt, B. Dudouet, S. Robine, and M. Dauça. 1987. Stage-specific polypeptides and villin expression during the intestinal epithelium substitution of the metamorphosing amphibian. *Differentiation* **36:** 116.

Glenney, J.R., N. Geisler, P. Kaulfus, and K. Weber. 1981. Demonstration of at least two different actin binding sites in villin in a calcium regulated modulator of F-actin organization. *J. Biol. Chem.* **256:** 8156.

Gröne, H.-J., K. Weber, U. Helmchen, and M. Osborn. 1986. Villin — A marker of brush border differentiation and cellular origin in human renal cell carcinoma. *Am. J. Pathol.* **124:** 294.

Maunoury, R., S. Robine, E. Pringault, C. Huet, J.L. Guénet, J.A. Gaillard, and D. Louvard. 1988. Villin expression in the visceral endoderm and in the gut anlage during early mouse embryogenesis. *EMBO J.* **7:** 3321.

Moll, R., S. Robine, B. Dudouet, and D. Louvard. 1987. Villin: A cytoskeletal protein and an early differentiation marker expressed in some human adenocarcinomas. *Virchows Arch. Cell Pathol.* **54:** 155.

Mooseker, M.S., T.A. Graves, K.A. Wharton, N. Falco, and C.L. Howe. 1980. Regulation of microvillus structure: Calcium-dependent solation and cross-linking of actin filaments in the microvilli of intestinal epithelial cells. *J. Cell Biol.* **87:** 809.

Reggio, H., E. Coudrier, and D. Louvard. 1982. Surface and cytoplasmic domains in polarized epithelial cells. In *Membrane in growth and development*, p. 89. A.R. Liss, New York.

Robine, S., C. Huet, R. Moll, C. Sahuquillo-Merino, E. Coudrier, A.

Zweibaum, and D. Louvard. 1985. Can villin be used to identify malignant and undifferentiated normal digestive epithelial cells? *Proc. Natl. Acad. Sci.* **82:** 8488.

West, A.B., C.A. Isaac, J.M. Carboni, J.S. Morrow, M.S. Mooseker, and K.W. Barwick. 1988. Localization of villin, a cytoskeletal protein specific to microvilli, in human ileum and colon and in in colonic neoplasms. *Gastroenterology* **94:** 343.

The Spectrin-based Cortical Cytoskeleton: A Role in Tumor Diagnosis?

J.S. Morrow, M. Younes, A.S. Harris, and P.E. Shile

Department of Pathology, Yale University School of Medicine,
New Haven, Connecticut 06510

Spectrins are a class of high-molecular-weight multifunctional actin-binding proteins associated with the cortical cytoplasm of most cells. They are distinguished by a number of shared activities and structural features (Table 1). The most studied member of this class is the protein purified from human erythrocyte ghosts. In the erythrocyte, the list of directly associated proteins includes protein 4.1, ankyrin, actin, adducin, and calmodulin. Other indirectly associated proteins include band 3, glycophorin, tropomyosin, a tropomyosin-binding protein, and probably many others that await discovery (for reviews, see Bennett 1985; Marchesi 1985; Morrow and Anderson 1986; Mische and Morrow 1988; T.C. Coleman et al., in prep.).

More recently, it has been recognized that all cells probably contain some form(s) of spectrin and that proteins of the spectrin family have a long evolutionary history. Coincident with these discoveries has been an understandable, if lamentable, confusion in the nomenclature. Names that have been used besides spectrin include fodrin, calspectin, calmodulin-binding protein, brain actin-binding protein (BABP), and TW260/240 (e.g., see Levine and Willard 1981; Sobue et al. 1982; Glenney et al. 1982). Gradually, most workers are now adapting the term spectrin for the generic class, prefixed with the tissue of origin and the designation α or β to signify the subunits. However, even this nomenclature is inadequate because the molecular weights of the subunits may vary; and even within subunits of the same relative molecular weight (by SDS-PAGE), there is increasing evidence for variability at the sequence and antigenic level. Additional confusion has also been engendered by comparisons between species. For example, the spectrin(s) in nucleated erythrocytes of nonmammalian (e.g., avian) species

Table 1 Features and Functions Associated with Mammalian Spectrin

α-Subunit	
molecular weight	240,000
number of known isoforms	2
length (nM)	97
number 106 residue units	21
binding role in heterodimer	β-subunit
	actin
	calmodulin
	CDP
β-Subunit	
molecular weights	220,000, 235,000
number of known isoforms	4
length (nM)	78–97
number 106 residue units	18+
binding role in heterodimer	α subunit
	protein 4.1
	calmodulin
	(in erythroid 220)
	ankyrin
	site of phosphorylation
	adducin
Other putative binding activities	intermediate filament
	microtubule
	synapsin I
	calpactin
	N-CAM
	GP-180

has features intermediate between those of mammalian erythroid and nonerythroid spectrin.

With the recognition of the nonerythroid spectrins has come a realization that their intracellular distribution and role may also be quite dissimilar from that in the erythrocyte. For example, spectrins have been found at the terminal web of the intestinal brush border (Glenney et al. 1982); with the Na,K-ATPase at the basolateral margins of kidney epithelial cells (Koob et al. 1987; Nelson and Veshnock 1987; Morrow et al. 1988); differentially segregated in axons and neurons (Lazarides and Nelson 1983; Zagon et al. 1986); with the acetylcholine receptor of skeletal muscle (Bloch and Morrow 1988); and in the cytoplasm, possibly associated with intracellular vesicular compartments (Black et al. 1988). The list of functions identified in vitro has also been extended (Table 1). If a unifying theme can be found in these emerging studies, one may speculate that the most general role of the spectrin cytoskeleton may be to organize topographically distinct receptor domains, possibly by controlling plasma membrane–vesicle traffic and/or by stabilizing existing receptor complexes (Perrin et al. 1987; Morrow et al. 1988; for review, see T.C. Coleman et al., in prep.). Coincident with this hypothesis, it appears that spectrin and its associated proteins are subject to many levels of posttranslational control (for review, see Mische and Morrow 1988).

Although the biology of spectrin continues to be an area of intense interest, whether an understanding of spectrin will be of value in tumor diagnosis or management is of equal interest. Certainly, there are a priori reasons to be optimistic. Spectrin is a relatively abundant protein, and several other cytoskeletal proteins discussed elsewhere in this volume have proved their value. However, this optimism must be weighed by the recognition that spectrin is a very large cytoplasmic protein that is relatively easily degraded during preparation and by the fact that relatively little is known about the diversity of spectrin isoforms. At this preliminary stage, it can be envisioned that three properties of spectrin may prove useful diagnostically: (1) the existence of unique tissue-specific isoforms; (2) the propensity to undergo specific posttranslational modifications that may accompany cell maturation; and (3) the changes in abundance or intracellular distribution that accompany neoplastic transformation.

Evidence for Tissue-specific Isoforms

Several isoforms of spectrin have been identified on the basis of antigenic or molecular-weight criteria (Table 2). Most of these arise due to species differences and therefore are of little diagnostic value. Restricting the discussion to mammalian forms, four subunits are widely recognized: α (240) and β (220) erythrocyte and α (240) and β (235) brain spectrin. Although the complete sequence of any subunit remains to be determined, existing structural and antigenic studies find about 50–60% homology between the erythroid and nonerythroid spectrin α-subunits and no significant differences in the nonerythroid spectrin (fodrin) from various tissues (or expression libraries) that have been examined. In addition, only a single copy of the α fodrin gene has been found (on chromosome 9) (Leto et al.

217

Table 2 Recognized Spectrin Isoforms

Spectrin isoform	Location	Composition[a]
1. Mammalian erythroid	erythrocyte	240/220
2. Avian erythroid	erythrocyte; muscle	240/230/220
3. Mammalian brain subtype 1	most nonerythroid	240/235
4. Mammalian brain subtype 2	dendrites; cell bodies	240/235E
5. Mammalian muscle subtype 1	acetylcholine receptors	220S
6. Avian brain subtype 1	most nonerythroid	240/235
7. Avian brain subtype 2	perikaryon; dendrites	240/220
8. Avian TW260/240	intestinal brush border	240/260
9. *Xenopus laevis*	egg; adult	240/?
10. *Drosophila*	S cells; embryo	234/226
11. Sea urchin	egg; embryo/sperm	237/234
12. *Dictyostelium*	amoebas	220/220
13. *Acanthamoeba*	amoebas	260

[a]As determined on SDS-PAGE, given in $M_r \times 10^{-3}$.

1988). Because most of the in vitro functions of spectrin can be attributed to the β-subunit (Table 1), it seems likely that this subunit might provide a potentially richer source of tissue diversity. Unfortunately, much less is known about the sequence of the β-subunit and almost nothing about the sequence of nonerythroid β. However, on the basis of antigenic criteria, it appears that at least four isoforms of β spectrin exist: the 220,000 M_r subunit of erythrocyte spectrin; the M_r 235,000 subunit of brain spectrin; a 235,000 M_r subunit (termed 235E) (Zagon et al. 1986) that is highly cross-reactive with erythrocyte β spectrin but is found in brain and skeletal muscle; and an M_r 220,000 spectrin (termed 220S) that shows limited cross-reactivity with erythrocyte β spectrin and is associated with the acetylcholine receptor in skeletal muscle (Bloch and Morrow 1988). This latter form may also be present in astrocytes.

In skeletal muscle, these isoforms demonstrate unique distributions. Polyclonal antibodies to brain α spectrin (240) or brain β spectrin (235) stain only the sarcolemma and (surrounding) endothelial cells. Most antibodies to erythrocyte spectrin (either α- or β-subunit, including a commercially obtained antibody to 235E spectrin), stain determinants overlying the Z-disks of sarcomeres. In addition, one polyclonal antibody to erythrocyte spectrin and MAbVIIF7, a monoclonal antibody directed to the β-I domain of erythrocyte β spectrin (Harris et al. 1986), stain the cytoplasmic face of motor endplates (Bloch and Morrow 1988). Fractionation of skeletal muscle homogenates in a 20–45% sucrose gradient, followed by immunoprecipitation, identifies immunoreactive spectrin peptides of M_r 240,000, 235,000, and 220,000. The 235,000 M_r subunit (235E) in the denser sucrose fractions (triads, cisternae, etc.) only precipitates with antierythrocyte spectrin antibodies. In separate experiments, MAbVIIF7 has been used to immunoprecipitate an M_r 220,000 spectrin subunit (220S) from isolated rat myotubes, and a colocalization of this subunit with the acetylcholine receptor has been identified (Bloch and Morrow 1988). In preliminary experiments, astrocytes in the hippocampus have also been found to stain for this same monoclonal antibody. These results suggest that there may indeed be distinct isoforms of spectrin that vary on a tissue-specific basis. The difficulty in identifying such isoforms antigenically may relate to their low abundance but may also simply mean that these tissue-specific spectrins vary only slightly from the predominant erythroid or nonerythroid spectrins. This variability probably arises due to alternate mRNA splicing, although much more information on the sequence of these proteins and the genes encoding them is needed before firm conclusions can be made.

Posttranslational Modification of Spectrin

A second feature of nonerythroid spectrin of potential diagnostic interest is its proteolysis by calcium-dependent proteases (CDPs). This does not appear to be a simple degradative event for several reasons: (1) The processing of brain spectrin at the synaptic junction is correlated with the development of long-term potentiation, and antibodies to brain spectrin block this event in vitro (Lynch and Baudry 1984); (2) a similar event appears to accompany cell activation in at least some other tissues (e.g., see Fox et al. 1987); (3) the proteolysis of brain spectrin is tightly regulated by calcium and calmodulin, such that calcium activates cleavage of the α-subunit by CDP at nearly the exact center of the molecule (Harris and Morrow 1988; Harris et al. 1988 and in prep.), whereas calmodulin regulates the susceptibility of the β-subunit by CDP-I; and (4) in vitro, CDP-I cleavage and calmodulin act synergistically to regulate the ability of brain spectrin to cross-link actin filaments. This

219

cleavage process can be easily detected by Western blot analysis, and the potential to prepare antibodies specific for either the processed or intact form of spectrin exists. Because CDP processing of some nonerythroid spectrins may accompany terminal differentiation, the state of spectrin processing may be of value in tumor analysis.

Changes in Spectrin Distribution and/or Abundance

In mature nonerythroid cells, the distribution of spectrin is often highly polarized, a feature lacking in immature cells (at least in culture). Thus, even without tissue specificity, the distribution and abundance of spectrin may be a useful marker of the state of "maturity" of a tumor. In MDCK cells in culture, the total abundance of spectrin falls as the cells approach confluence, and the cytoplasmic spectrin distribution characteristic of nonconfluent cells gives way to a basolateral distribution. A similar phenomenon appears to occur in the transition from normal colonic epithelium to neoplastic epithelium. Cells of colonic adenomas and carcinomas have two to three times more spectrin per weight of total protein, and the distribution of this spectrin becomes more diffuse on the cell surface and in the cytoplasm. Such an increase in other cytoskeletal proteins, such as villin, is not so apparent. It remains to be determined whether these changes will be of value in detecting precancer or in aiding the diagnosis of small biopsies and/or cytologic specimens.

SUMMARY

The spectrin-based cortical cytoskeleton is emerging as one of the primary mechanisms by which a cell establishes and maintains the topographic organization of its plasma membrane. Because such organization is a hallmark of the differentiated state, the study of spectrin may offer unique tools for the evaluation of tumors. Before this can become a practical reality, significant obstacles must be overcome. Tissue-specific isoforms of spectrin clearly exist, although it is likely that, with some exceptions, they will differ from each other in only very limited ways. Therefore, sequence information is needed, so that peptide-specific antibodies and hybridization probes can be prepared. In addition, their cytoplasmic location and sensitivity to degradation makes them more difficult to evaluate, especially given that the distribution of spectrin and its quantity may be useful information.

REFERENCES

Bennett, V. 1985. The membrane skeleton of human erythrocytes and its implications for more complex cells. *Annu. Rev. Biochem.* **54:** 273.

Black, J.D., S.T. Koury, R.B. Bankert, and E.A. Repasky. 1988. Heterogeneity in lymphocyte spectrin distribution: Ultrastructural identification of a new spectrin-rich cytoplasmic structure. *J. Cell Biol.* **106:** 97.

Bloch, R.J. and J.S. Morrow. 1988. An unusual beta spectrin associated with clustered acetylcholine receptors. *J. Cell Biol.* (in press).

Fox, J.E.B., C.C. Reynolds, J.S. Morrow, and D.R. Phillips. 1987. Spectrin is associated with membrane-bound actin filaments in platelets and is hydrolyzed by the Ca dependent protease during platelet activation. *Blood* **69:** 537.

Glenney, J.R., Jr., P. Glenney, M. Osborn, and K. Weber. 1982. An F-actin and calmodulin binding protein from isolated intestinal brush borders has a morphology related to spectrin. *Cell* **28:** 843.

Harris, A.S. and J.S. Morrow. 1988. Proteolytic processing of human brain alpha spectrin (fodrin): Identification of a hypersensitive site. *J. Neurosci.* **8:** 2640.

Harris, A.S., D.E. Croall, and J.S. Morrow. 1988. The calmodulin binding site in alpha fodrin is near the calcium-dependent protease-I cleavage site. *J. Biol. Chem.* **263:** 15754.

Harris, A.S., J.P. Anderson, P.D. Yurchenco, L.A.D. Green, K.J. Ainger, and J.S. Morrow. 1986. Mechanisms of cytoskeletal regulation: Functional and antigenic diversity in human erythrocyte and brain beta spectrin. *J. Cell. Biochem.* **30:** 51.

Koob, R., M. Zimmermann, W. Schoner, and D. Drenckhahn. 1987. Colocalization and coprecipitation of ankyrin and Na,K-ATPase in kidney epithelial cells. *Eur. J. Cell Biol.* **45:** 230.

Lazarides, E., and W.J. Nelson. 1983. Erythrocyte and brain forms of spectrin in the cerebellum form distinct membrane-cytoskeletal domains in neurons. *Science* **220:** 1295.

Leto, T.L., D. Fortugno-Erikson, D. Barton, T.L. Yang-Feng, U. Francke, A.S. Harris, J.S. Morrow, V.T. Marchesi, and E.J. Benz. 1988. Comparison of nonerythroid alpha spectrin genes reveals strict homology among diverse species. *Mol. Cell. Biol.* **8:** 1.

Levine, J., and M. Willard. 1981. Fodrin: An axonally transported polypeptide associated with the internal periphery of many cells. *J. Cell Biol.* **90:** 631.

Lynch, G. and M. Baudry. 1984. The biochemistry of memory: A new and specific hypothesis. *Science* **224:** 1057.

Marchesi, V.T. 1985. Stabilizing infrastructure of cell membranes. *Annu. Rev. Cell Biol.* **1:** 531.

Mische, S.M. and J.S. Morrow. 1988. Post-translational regulation of the erythrocyte cortical cytoskeleton. *Protoplasma* **145:** 167.

Morrow, J.S. and R.A. Anderson. 1986. Shaping the too fluid bilayer. *Lab. Invest.* **54:** 237.

Morrow, J.S., C.D. Cianci, T. Ardito, A.S. Mann, and M. Kashgarian. 1988. Ankyrin links fodrin to the alpha subunit of Na,K-ATPase in Madin-Darby canine kidney cells and in intact renal tubule cells. *J. Cell Biol.* (in press).

Nelson, W.J. and P.I. Veshnock. 1987. Ankyrin binding to Na,K-ATPase and implications for the organization of membrane domains in polarized cells. *Nature* **328**: 533.

Perrin, D., O.K. Langley, and D. Aunis. 1987. Anti-alpha-fodrin inhibits secretion from permeabilized chromaffin cells. *Nature* **326**: 498.

Sobue, D.L., K. Kanda, M. Inui, K. Morimoto, and S. Kakiuchi. 1982. Actin polymerization induced by calspectin, a calmodulin-binding spectrin like protein. *FEBS Lett.* **148**: 221.

Zagon, I.S., R. Higbee, B.M. Riederer, and S.R. Goodman. 1986. Spectrin subtypes in mammalian brain: An immunoelectron microscopic study. *J. Neurosci.* **6**: 2977.

Diagnostic Cytology and Cell Markers: Some Practical Considerations

L.G. Koss

Department of Pathology, Montefiore Medical Center
Albert Einstein College of Medicine, Bronx, New York 10467

Diagnostic cytology is the branch of human pathology dealing with interpretations of cell samples in the diagnosis of human diseases. Although a broad variety of infections and degenerative disorders may be so identified, the principal targets of diagnostic cytology are detection and diagnosis of precancerous states and of cancer.

Cancer Detection

The target organs of cytologic cancer detection systems are listed in Table 1. Precancerous states and early cancer are recognized by cell changes affecting primarily the nucleus of the epithelial cells and, to a lesser extent, the cytoplasm. Because the type and configuration of the target epithelia is well known, cell markers are rarely needed for diagnosis, if ever.

The detection of precancerous states, however, poses its own problems. For example, the ratio of detected precancerous states of the uterine cervix to invasive cancer strongly suggests that only a fraction of the intraepithelial abnormalities, probably not more than 10%, progress to invasive cancer. The progressing lesions cannot be distinguished by morphology or DNA ploidy analysis from stationary or regressing lesions. Within recent years, the role of human papillomavirus (HPV)

Table 1 Target Organs for Cancer Detection by Cytologic Techniques

Female genital tract	Lower urinary tract
uterine cervix	bladder
vagina	ureter and renal pelvis
endometrium	
ovary and tube	
Respiratory tract	Gastrointestinal tract
oral cavity	esophagus
larynx	stomach
bronchus	colon

223

as a factor in the genesis of precancerous lesions of the genital tract has been suggested (see Syrjanen et al. 1987). The possibility that HPV types 16, 18, and 31 are more commonly associated with progression than types 6 and 11 is based so far on indirect evidence, including in situ hybridization of viral DNA and RNA. This "guilt by association" is mitigated by the observation that HPV infection, including HPV types 16 and 18, is common in populations at large (De Villiers et al. 1987). Hence, if the presence of "high-risk" HPV were to be used as a marker of disease, cancerophobia would become a widespread social disorder.

There is an obvious need for additional markers that could be used as predictors of the progression of precancerous states. Recently, we studied the possible role of Harvey (Ha)-*ras* oncogene expression in gastric cancer with interesting results suggestive of two different pathways of gastric cancer genesis (B. Czerniak et al., in prep.).

Cancer Diagnosis

In reference to cancer diagnosis, the scope of cytology comprises virtually all organs (Koss 1979). Thus, samples of various fluids, such as voided urine sputum and effusions, are a common target of cytologic diagnoses. The thin-needle aspiration biopsy is a method of diagnosis that is applicable to a broad variety of situations affecting all organs (Koss et al. 1984). This method is inexpensive, rapid, and, in experienced hands, quite accurate.

The problems that must be considered in cytologic diagnoses are as follows: (1) Is the lesion a cancer or not? (2) If the lesion is benign, can its cause be identified? (3) If the lesion is malignant, what is the type and origin? (4) Is the lesion curable and, if so, what is the best therapy? In the presence of an accurate clinical history and an adequate cytologic sample, these questions can usually be answered. There are, however, some situations where the use of markers is justified. Several examples are listed in Table 2.

Many attempts have been made to identify intermediate filaments as specific markers that would differentiate mesothelial cells of mesenchymal origin from epithelial cells of epidermal or endodermal origin. These attempts have not been fully successful to date. The likely reason is that all cells have, at birth, a full complement of structural genes and that the activation of these genes follows pathways that are not fully un-

Table 2 Examples of Diagnostic Situations Wherein Cell Markers Are Useful

Source of cells	Target of differential diagnosis
Effusions	mesothelial cells and macrophages vs. cancer cells carcinoma vs. mesothelioma small cell carcinoma vs. lymphoma primary site of origin of metastatic cancer
Lung	undifferentiated large cell carcinoma vs. adenocarcinoma
Cervix	undifferentiated epidermoid carcinoma vs. adenocarcinoma
Aspiration biopsy	small cell carcinoma vs. lymphoma carcinoma vs. melanoma carcinoma vs. soft part sarcoma primary site of origin of metastatic cancer

derstood at this time. Thus, keratin expression is common to all epithelia regardless of embryonal derivation, whereas vimentin is expressed sometimes and not at other times. Desmin, on the other hand, is difficult to demonstrate in our hands. Still, successful application of monoclonal antibodies to intermediate filaments in classification of tumors in aspiration biopsy material has been reported repeatedly (Osborn and Weber 1983; Domagala et al. 1986a,b, 1988).

The use of tumor-specific markers, particularly in aspiration biopsy material, is perhaps somewhat easier than the use of cell differentiation markers. Some examples are shown in Table 3.

Table 3 Some Tumor-specific Markers Applicable to Cytology

Markers	Tumors most likely to carry the markers
Estrogen and progesteron receptors	mammary carcinoma; endometrial carcinoma
Polypeptide hormones	endocrine tumors; various 1° sites; occasional ectopic secretion by other tumors
Human chorionic gonadotrophin	trophoblastic neoplasia; germ cell tumors
Glial fibrillary acidic proteins	tumors of glial origin

225

Calcitonin staining, using the appropriate monoclonal antibody, was helpful in several instances in the identification of a poorly differentiated medullary carcinoma of the thyroid and human chorionic gonadotropin in the identification of a mediastinal teratoma with a component of choricarcinoma.

Prognostic Assessment of Human Cancer
Cell markers can also be used for a possible prognostic assessment of various human cancers. Some of the measurable cell markers in tumor prognosis are (1) DNA measurements, (2) oncogene expression, and (3) epidermal growth factor receptors.

By far, the most common approach to tumor prognostication is the measurement of DNA, using either flow cytometry or image cytophotometry (Koss et al. 1988). Flow cytometry requires a preparation of a suspension of single cells or nuclei and staining with a fluorescent probe that binds stoichiometrically to double-stranded DNA, e.g., propidium iodide or ethidium bromide. Image cytophotometry requires the use of a Feulgen reaction, which stains DNA. These measurements are based on the assumption that differences in DNA ploidy values reflect the genetic makeup of the tumor, with diploid tumors likely to exhibit a less aggressive behavior than aneuploid tumors.

This hypothesis has been proved correct to a significant extent in some tumors and in some organ systems, such as tumors of the prostate and the urinary bladder urothelium (Koss and Greenebaum 1986). For most tumors and organ systems, however, the prognostic value of DNA measurements has either not been proved or does not apply. Carcinomas of the thyroid, for example, are often diploid and are still capable of metastases.

The use of cell markers finds an interesting applicability in flow cytometry, as it may allow the separation of cells of one specific origin from cells of other derivation by appropriate gating. The measurements of the DNA may thus be performed on a cell population that is better defined. As an example, staining for keratin filaments may be used to identify epithelial cells in bladder washings. DNA measurements on this discrete cell population may disclose abnormalities of DNA content that were not evident when the entire specimen was examined (Feitz et al. 1985). Markers for subpopulations of lymphocytes may also be helpful in this regard.

Other approaches to prognostication include oncogene expression that may be quantitated by image analysis of cells stained with an antibody to a protein product such as p21. The analysis is performed on peroxidase/antiperoxidase-stained cell preparations, and histograms of light absorption at the appropriate wave length are constructed. The oncogene products can also be measured by flow cytometry in experimental cell systems. Although some data suggest that oncogene expression may be of prognostic value, the issue cannot be considered as settled.

It is quite clear from this brief review that there are many issues with the use of cell markers in diagnostic cytology that require additional research. Perhaps the most important issue is the need for simple, uncomplicated laboratory methods that would allow for a clear persuasive staining of routine, usually alcohol-fixed, material. The peroxidase/antiperoxidase routine often fails under these circumstances. The cell permeabilization routine must also be standardized. In my experience, the application of markers in routine diagnostic cytology is much more difficult than in tissue pathology, and false positive and false negative results are not uncommon.

REFERENCES

Domagala, W., K. Weber, and M. Osborn. 1986a. Differential diagnosis of lymph node aspirates by intermediate filament typing of tumor cells. *Acta Cytol.* **30:** 225.

———. 1988. Diagnostic significance of coexpression of intermediate filaments in fine needle aspirates of human tumors. *Acta Cytol.* **32:** 49.

Domagala, W., J. Lubinski, K. Weber, and M. Osborn. 1986b. Intermediate filament typing of tumor cells in fine needle aspirates by means of monoclonal antibodies. *Acta Cytol.* **30:** 214.

De Villiers, E.M., D. Wagner, A. Schneider, H. Wesch, H. Miklaw, J. Wahrendorf, U. Papendick, and H. zur Hausen. 1987. Human papillomavirus infections in women with and without abnormal cervical cytology. *Lancet* **II:** 703.

Feitz, W.F.J., H.L.M. Beck, A.W.G.B. Smeets, F.M.J. Debruyne, G.P. Vooijs, C.J. Herman, and F.C.S. Ramaekers. 1985. Tissue-specific markers in flow cytometry of urological cancers: Cytokeratins in bladder carcinoma. *Int. J. Cancer* **36:** 349.

Koss, L.G. 1979. *Diagnostic cytology and its histopathologic bases,* 3rd edition. J.B. Lippincott, Philadelphia.

Koss, L.G. and E. Greenebaum. 1986. Measuring DNA in human cancer. *J. Am. Med. Assoc.* **255:** 3158.

Koss, L.G., S. Wyoke, and W. Olszewski. 1984. *Aspiration biopsy. Cytologic interpretation and histologic bases.* Igaku Shoin, Tokyo.

Koss, L.G., B. Czerniak, F. Herz, and R.R. Wersto. 1988. Flow cytometric measurements of DNA and other cell components in human tumors. A critical appraisal. *Hum. Pathol.* (in press).

Osborn, M. and K. Weber. 1983. Tumor diagnosis by intermediate fila-ment typing. *Lab. Invest.* **48:** 372.

Syrjanen, K., L. Gissman, and L.G. Koss, eds. 1987. *Papillomaviruses and human disease*. Springer-Verlag, Berlin.

Intermediate Filament Typing as a Diagnostic Aid in Fine-needle Aspiration Cytology

M. Osborn[1] and W. Domagala[1,2]

[1]Max Planck Institute for Biophysical Chemistry
D-3400 Göttingen, Federal Republic of Germany

[2]Department of Tumor Pathology, Medical Academy
Szczecin, Poland

Advantages of using cytoskeletal proteins as an adjunct in histological classification include the following: (1) Such proteins are usually well understood at a protein chemical level, and most have also been characterized in cell biological studies. (2) They are often major cellular constituents, e.g., actin and intermediate filaments (IFs). Thus, their presence may be expected to influence the appearance of the cytoplasm. (3) If the differential diagnostic question is appropriately formulated, use of antibodies to cytoskeletal proteins can give an unambiguous answer in some situations that are difficult to decide by conventional staining methods such as hematoxylin-eosin. Such methods are of particular importance if there are no perceptible signs of differentiation at the light microscope level.

Here, we concentrate on studies designed to assess the use of antibodies specific for the different types of IFs in routine cytological diagnosis. We have concentrated on fine-needle aspiration (FNA) biopsy smears, which form an increasingly important part of cytological material, but the methods used are equally applicable to exfoliative cytology (sputum, body cavity effusions, touch imprints, brushes, cerebral spinal fluid, urine, or bone marrow smears). Routine cytology has the further advantage that the method used to fix the samples—for our material immersion in 96% ethanol—is optimal for the assay of IF proteins by immunocytochemistry and employs the same methods originally used to visualize IFs in cell lines. Our results suggest that when the clinical information and morphology of the tumor cells are used to frame the diagnostic question, IF typing can often refine the cytologic diagnosis of major tumor types and can help prevent error in certain situations (Altmannsberger et al. 1984; Droese et al. 1984; Domagala et al. 1986a,b, 1987b, 1988b,c). It seems to be of particular value in difficult cases where no unambiguous diagnosis of tumor type can be provided from consideration of the clinical information and the morphology at the light microscope level, but of course, it does not resolve all such cases.

Antibodies
Most of the IF antibodies used in this study are available commercially. As broad specificity keratin antibodies, we used the monoclonal antibody KL1 isolated by J. Viac et al. and lu5 isolated by J. von Overbeck. Other monoclonal antibodies isolated in our laboratory include V9 for vimentin; DEB5 or DER11 for desmin, NR4, which sees neurofilament-low (NF-L); NN18, which sees NF-M (middle); and NE52, which sees phosphorylated and unphosphorylated forms of NF-H (high), for neurofilaments; and GA-5 for glial fibrillary acidic protein. In addition, in some experiments, we have used chain-specific keratin antibodies to detect whether single keratin polypeptides are present, as well as a commercial leukocyte common antigen antibody. Specificity of a particular antibody has been usually documented by immunoblotting and by using it on normal human tissues where the distribution of different cell types is known.

Cytological Specimens
Conventional FNA biopsy is quite accurate in distinguishing benign from malignant lesions (Droese et al. 1984; Koss et al. 1984). If the tumor cells show easily recognizable features at the light microscope level, these features can be recognized by a trained cytologist, and a specific cytological diagnosis can be provided. We have examined 271 such cases collected at random (group A) and compared the results obtained by conventional cytology, IF typing of the FNA biopsy smears, and subsequent histology of the tumors (Domagala et al. 1988c). Our results with this group show that IF typing confirmed the specific cytological diagnosis of major tumor types in 97% of these cases and changed it in 3% of the cases. The most common change was from initial diagnosis of anaplastic carcinoma to one of malignant lymphoma, once the immunological and histologic results were known.

Analysis of the group A cases further confirmed the IF con-

Table 1 IF Typing of FNA – Carcinomas

Origin	No. of cases	Keratin	Vimentin	NF
Merkel cell	9	9/9	0/9	9/9
Thyroid, medullary	2	2/2	2/2	2/2
Thyroid (P,F,LC), kidney, endometrium, ovary	39	39/39	37/39	
Lung-Sc	12	12/12	2/12	
Breast	28	28/28	3/18	
Adrenal, prostate, larnyx (SC)	10	10/10	3/10	
SC (lung, skin, esophagus, uterus, cervix)	20	22/22	0/13	
AdC (stomach, pancreas, L-bowel, liver)	23	23/23	0/20	
Primary not known	63	63/63	7/46	
Total	206			

(P) Papillary; (F) follicular; (LC) large cell; (SC) squamous cell carcinoma; (Sc) small cell; (Adc) adenocarcinoma; (L) large.

tent expected from previous results on IF expression in histological sections of the same tumor type and also allowed an assessment of the frequency of coexpression of keratin and vimentin in carcinomas from different sites. In many instances, this was performed by double-label immunofluorescence microscopy, using keratin and vimentin antibodies. As seen in Table 1, carcinomas at certain sites such as thyroid, kidney, endometrium, and ovary very often show coexpression of keratin and vimentin in the majority of cases and tumor cells (Domagala et al. 1988a,d). Carcinomas at other sites such as breast show coexpression of keratin and vimentin in some cells in a few instances, whereas coexpression has not been observed in the carcinomas of the gastrointestinal tract. Merkel cell carcinomas coexpress keratin and neurofilament polypeptides. The IF distribution in this tumor is so characteristic that the buttons of IF filaments, which often remain attached to the otherwise bare nucleus, provide an additional criteria helpful in the differential diagnosis of this tumor in conventionally stained FNA smears (Domagala et al. 1987a).

The second group of cases analyzed were preselected as difficult cases in which an unambiguous cytologic diagnosis of major tumor type could not be provided by conventional stains and by consideration of the clinical data (Domagala et al. 1988c). These cases lack early visible signs of differentiation at the light microscope level. This second group, group B, was also subjected to IF typing of the FNA biopsy smear, and subsequent histology of each tumor was also performed. In group B, IF typing confirmed the cytological suggestion of major tumor type in 38% of the cases, changed it in 7%, helped resolve ambiguities in 45%, and was of no help in 10%. Again, the most frequent diagnostic dilemma in which IF typing was instrumental in changing the diagnosis was to decide between anaplastic carcinoma and malignant lymphoma. Where the cytologic suggestion was malignant carcinoma or malignant lymphoma, IF typing provided data favoring a diagnosis of carcinoma in 6 of 28 cases and a diagnosis of malignant lymphoma in 22 of 28 cases. IF typing was also clearly of use in further refining the diagnosis in small, round cell tumors of children. It did not help in other instances. For example, IF typing cannot help in deciding between sarcoma and malignant melanoma (both V+) and did not help when the diagnosis required a decision between seminoma and embryonal carcinoma.

In comparison with the much greater amount of data available from IF typing of histological sections of human tumors, relatively few cases have been examined in cytology by relatively few laboratories. As in histology, a set of antibodies against the different IF proteins can yield more information and build more confidence in the method than the selection of only a single IF antibody. Our own results, as well as the increasing use of these methods by others (Ramaekers et al. 1984; for overview, see Goerttler et al. 1988), encourage the idea that IF typing has a role to play in routine cytological diagnosis. Obviously, other antibodies such as chain-specific keratin antibodies, leukocyte common antigen, epithelial membrane antigen, syneptophysin, and so forth, can be employed to yield further information valuable in classification of major tumor types in FNA cytology. However, such methods are only likely to be successful when the clinical information and light microscopy are used to first formulate the diagnostic question and when the conventional light microscopy and the immunological results are interpreted by the same cytopathologist.

REFERENCES
Altmannsberger, M., M. Osborn, M. Droese, K. Weber, and A. Schauer. 1984. Diagnostic value of intermediate filament antibodies in clinical cytology. *Klin. Wochenschr.* **62:** 114.

Domagala, W., K. Weber, and M. Osborn. 1986a. Differential diagnosis of lymph node aspirates by intermediate filament typing of tumor cells. *Acta Cytol.* **30:** 225.

————. 1988a. Diagnostic significance of coexpression of intermediate filaments in fine needle aspirates of human tumors. *Acta Cytol.* **32:** 49.

Domagala, W., J. Lubinski, K. Weber, and M. Osborn. 1986b. Intermediate filament typing of tumor cells in fine needle aspirates using monoclonal antibodies. *Acta Cytol.* **30:** 214.

————. 1988b. Intermediate filament typing vs. electron microscopy in the diagnosis of major tumor types in fine needle aspirates. In *New frontiers in cytology* (ed. K. Goerttler et al.). Springer Verlag, Berlin.

Domagala, W., J. Lasota, M. Chosia, A. Szadowska, K. Weber, and M. Osborn. 1988c. Diagnosis of major tumor categories in fine needle aspirates is more accurate when light microscopy is combined with intermediate filament typing: A study of 403 cases. *Cancer* (in press).

Domagala, W., J. Lasota, H. Wolska, J. Lubinski, K. Weber, and M. Osborn. 1988d. Diagnosis of matastatic renal cell and thyroid carcinoma by intermediate filament typing and cytology of tumor cells in fine needle aspirates. *Acta Cytol.* **32:** 415.

Domagala, W., J. Lubinski, J. Lasota, I. Giryn, K. Weber, and M. Osborn. 1987a. Neuroendocrine (Merkel cell) skin carcinoma: Cytology, intermediate filament typing and ultrastructure of tumor cells in fine needle aspirates. *Acta Cytol.* **31:** 267.

Domagala, W., J. Lubinski, J. Lasota, S. Woyke, L. Wozniak, A. Szadowska, K. Weber, and M. Osborn. 1987b. Decisive role of intermediate filament typing of tumor cells in differential diagnosis of difficult fine needle aspirates. *Acta Cytol.* **31:** 253.

Droese, M., M. Altmannsberger, A. Kehl, P.G. Lankisch, R. Weiss, K. Weber, and M. Osborn. 1984. Ultrasound-guided percutaneous fine needle aspiration biopsy of abdominal and retroperitoneal masses: Accuracy of cytology in the diagnosis of malignancy, cytologic tumor typing and use of antibodies to intermediate filaments in selected cases. *Acta Cytol.* **28:** 368.

Goerttler, K., G.E. Feichter, and S. Witte, eds. 1988. *New frontiers in cytology.* Springer Verlag, Berlin.

Koss, L.G., S. Woyke, and W. Olszewski. 1984. *Aspiration biopsy: Cytologic interpretation and histologic bases.* Igaku Shoin, New York.

Ramaekers, F., D. Haag, P. Jap, and P.G. Vooijs. 1984. Immunochemical demonstration of keratin and vimentin in cytologic aspirates. *Acta Cytol.* **28:** 385.

Antibodies to Intermediate Filament Proteins as Tissue-specific Probes in the Flow Cytometric Analysis of Disease

F.C.S. Ramaekers, J.L.M. Beck, and G.P. Vooijs

Department of Pathology, University Hospital Nijmegen,
6525 GA Nijmegen, The Netherlands

Flow cytometric analysis of cell suspensions has proved to be a useful technique for the estimation and quantitation of several cellular components. Special attention has focused on the measurement of DNA content in cells, which may be used to estimate ploidy and proliferative capacity of tumors. However, analysis of mixed cell populations, which are normally obtained from tumors, gives rise to data that are sometimes difficult to interpret. Tumor cell suspensions usually contain variable amounts of other cell types, such as inflammatory and stromal cells. We have developed a flow cytometric procedure to distinguish epithelial, primarily tumor, cells from nonepithelial cells in such mixed cell populations on the basis of their intermediate filament content. With this method, it is possible to analyze simultaneously the DNA content and distribution of the two cell populations. After our earlier studies with a model system of mixed cultured cells (Ramaekers et al. 1984, 1986), we review our observations with cell suspensions from gynecological and urological tumors, with tumor cells present in body cavity fluids, and our studies on benign skin lesions. When cells isolated from normal endometrium and neoplastic lesions of the endometrium were fixed in 70% ethanol, stained for cytokeratin and DNA, and analyzed by flow cytometry, several cell populations could be distinguished. Cells positive for cytokeratin can be distinguished clearly from negative cells. Furthermore, propidium iodide (PI) staining distinguishes cells containing nuclei from cell debris and loose cytoplasmic fragments. A DNA histogram of the cytokeratin-positive cells can be obtained readily from these data by placing a window around these cells. The correctness of the window was checked by sorting samples of cells onto glass slides and by examination of these preparations in the fluorescence microscope and after

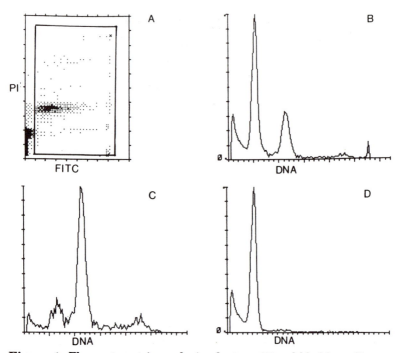

Figure 1 Flow cytometric analysis of a transitional bladder cell carcinoma in suspension after labeling for cytokeratin using a polyclonal keratin antiserum (FITC channel) and staining with PI. (*A*) Two parameter (FITC for cytokeratin and PI for DNA) analysis, showing position of the window containing epithelial cytokeratin-positive cells. The cytokeratin-negative, aneuploid fraction is represented by naked nuclei, as judged from microscopical observations. (*B*) DNA histogram of the total cell suspension. (*C*) DNA histogram of cytokeratin-positive cells selected by placing a window, as illustrated in *A*. The DNA index of the tumor cells was 1.83. (*D*) DNA histogram of cytokeratin-negative cells.

routine cytological staining. In these sorted samples, only cytokeratin- and PI-positive cells were found, in contrast to unsorted cell suspensions. Furthermore, cell morphology was well preserved and indicated the presence of mainly (if not only) epithelial (tumor) cells (Oud et al. 1985).

When similar cell suspensions from bladder transitional cell carcinomas and renal cell carcinomas were incubated with polyclonal or monoclonal cytokeratin antisera and thereafter with an appropriate FITC-conjugated second antibody and PI, again the carcinoma cells could be separated from stromal and inflammatory cells (Fig. 1). However, as can be judged from

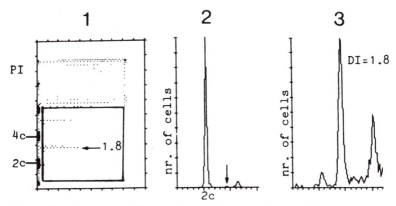

Figure 2 Flow cytometric analysis of an ovarian carcinoma present in ascites fluid. (*1*) Two-parameter analysis after labeling of the cells for cytokeratin. Cytokeratin-positive tumor cells are seen with a DNA index of 1.8. (*2*) DNA histogram of total cell population present in ascites. (*3*) Cytokeratin-positive tumor cells, which were not seen in *2* (arrow), are clearly detectable.

Figure 1, A and D, a cytokeratin-negative, aneuploid fraction is often present in these cell suspensions. We have sorted this population and, after microscopical inspection, concluded that it represents naked nuclei, which always occur in enzymatically or mechanically obtained cell suspensions from solid tumors. After comparing several DNA profiles of labeled and unlabeled cells, we further conclude that this phenomenon has no significant impact on the DNA distribution histograms of the tumor. Analysis of the cytokeratin and PI-positive bladder cells revealed tumor cells ranging in DNA index from 0.94 to 2.02 (normal human diploid equals 1.0). In addition, in cell suspensions from carcinomas in which very few tumor cells are recognized by one-dimensional DNA flow cytometry, double labeling allows cytokeratin-positive, aneuploid tumor cells to be distinguished clearly from the stromal cells and also from the cytokeratin-positive, but diploid, bladder and kidney epithelial cells (Feitz et al. 1985, 1986). In some cases, labeling of the renal carcinoma cells with the antiserum to vimentin revealed an FITC-positive aneuploid subpopulation of cells, in addition to diploid renal cells, stromal, and inflammatory components.

Application of keratin and vimentin antibodies in the flow cytometric analysis of body cavity effusions revealed that the double-labeling assay can significantly increase the level of tumor cell detection. Figure 2 illustrates such a flow cytometric analysis of an adenocarcinoma metastasis, present in

237

ascites. In this case, as well as in several other cases of tumor cells present in body cavity fluids that we have studied, the routinely obtained flow cytogram after PI labeling predominantly showed a diploid peak, representing mostly blood cells. In the case shown in Figure 2, a minor aneuploid peak could be discerned (arrow); but in many of the effusions examined in such a way, this was not the case. When cells from these effusions were labeled with a broadly cross-reacting monoclonal cytokeratin antibody and analyzed in a two-dimensional flow cytometric procedure, the carcinoma cells could clearly be distinguished in several cases.

Intermediate filament antibodies, in combination with flow cytometry, can also be helpful in the study of skin disease, e.g., in quantitative population analyses of healthy epidermis, psoriatic uninvolved epidermis, and psoriatic lesions. Using an antibody that stains only keratinizing cells and does not react with the basal cells in the tissues mentioned before (RKSE 60), we could show an almost sixfold increase in the germinative fraction in the psoriatic lesion. More interesting, the germinative fraction in psoriatic uninvolved epidermis was also significantly higher than normal (Bauer et al. 1986).

DISCUSSION

Flow cytometric analysis of mixed cell populations, such as those obtained from tumors, produces results that are often difficult to interpret because of the variable mixture of cells of interest, usually carcinoma cells, with other cells such as inflammatory and stromal cells.

Because of the ubiquitous presence of cell-type-specific intermediate filaments, immunofluorescence of these structures can be used for flow cytometric analysis of many solid tumors. All carcinomas can be distinguished from nonepithelial cells by broad-spectrum cytokeratin antibodies, and adenocarcinoma cells from nonglandular epithelial and nonepithelial elements by antibodies specific for glandular cells (Ramaekers et al. 1983). Two advantages of the application of cytokeratin antibodies in such selection procedures have become obvious in the present experiments.

First, in those cases of carcinomas where an aneuploid tumor cell peak could be detected in the one-dimensional DNA profile, labeling of the epithelial tumor cells with FITC for cytokeratin allowed the analysis of the DNA distribution in the tumor and estimation of its proliferative fraction separately from the stromal and inflammatory components. Second, in those tumor fractions where the malignant cells represent only a small fraction of the cells in suspension and thus cannot be recognized in the one-parameter analysis, labeling of the cells in suspension clearly displays such minor fractions in a two-parameter analysis, allowing the estimation of their ploidy and proliferative fractions.

REFERENCES

Bauer, F.W., J.B. Boezeman, M.S. van Engelen, R.M. de Grood, and F.C.S. Ramaekers. 1986. Monoclonal antibodies for epidermal population analysis. *J. Invest. Dermatol.* **87**: 72.

Feitz, W.F.J., H.L.M. Beck, A.W.G.B. Smeets, F.M.J. Debruyne, G.P. Vooijs, C.J. Herman, and F.C.S. Ramaekers. 1985. Tissue specific markers in flow cytometry of urological cancers: Cytokeratins in bladder carcinoma. *Int. J. Cancer* **36**: 349.

Feitz, W.F.J., H.F.M. Karthaus, H.L.M. Beck, J.C. Romijn, A.P.M. van der Meyden, F.M.J. Debruyne, G.P. Vooijs, and F.C.S. Ramaekers. 1986. Tissue specific markers in flow cytometry of urological cancers. II. Cytokeratin and vimentin in renal cell tumors. *Int. J. Cancer* **37**: 201.

Oud, P.S., J.B.J. Henderik, H.L.M. Beck, J.A.M. Veldhuizen, G.P. Vooijs, C.J. Herman, and F.C.S. Ramaekers. 1985. Flow cytometric analysis and sorting of human endometrial cells after immunocytochemical labeling for cytokeratin using a monoclonal antibody. *Cytometry* **6**: 159.

Ramaekers, F.C.S., H. Beck, G.P. Vooijs, and C.J. Herman. 1984. Flow-cytometric analysis of mixed cell populations using intermediate filament antibodies. *Exp. Cell Res.* **153**: 249.

Ramaekers, F.C.S., H.L.M. Beck, W.F.J. Feitz, P.S. Oud, F.M.J. Debruyne, G.P. Vooijs, and C.J. Herman. 1986. Application of antibodies to intermediate filament proteins as tissue-specific probes in the flow cytometric analysis of complex tumors. *Anal. Quant. Cytol. Histol.* **8**: 271.

Ramaekers, F.C.S., A. Huysmans, O. Moesker, A. Kant, P.H.K. Jap, C. Herman, and G.P. Vooijs. 1983. Monoclonal antibodies to keratin filaments, specific for glandular epithelia and their tumors. Use in surgical pathology. *Lab. Invest.* **49**: 353.

Micrometastasis: Characterization and Tumorigenicity of Disseminated Tumor Cells in Human Bone Marrow

I. Funke, G. Schlimok,[1] B. Bock, B. Schweiberer, and G. Riethmüller

Institut für Immunologie, Universität München, D-8000 Munich 2, Federal Republic of Germany

[1]Zentralklinikum Augsburg D-8900 Augsburg, Federal Republic of Germany

Early metastasis is the major cause of death from cancer in the western world. This is exemplified in breast and colorectal cancer, where up to one third of the patients already suffer from a disseminated cancer when their primary tumor is diagnosed. Thus, every effort appears to be warranted to define more accurately the stage of micrometastasis by direct identification of disseminated tumor cells before they have developed into established, incurable macrometastases. We have made use of the exquisite tissue specificity of cytokeratins to identify single disseminated cancer cells in patients with mammary, colorectal, and gastric cancer. Applying a monoclonal antibody specific for cytokeratin polypeptide 18 (Debus et al. 1982; antibody CK2, Boehringer-Mannheim GmbH), together with a sensitive alkaline phosphatase technique (APAAP) for the immunocytochemical detection of cytokeratin-positive cells, we have thus far analyzed 500 patients with the three groups of cancers mentioned. Depending on the tumor size, the involvement of regional lymph nodes, the presence of distant metastasis, the histological type, and the site of the primary tumor, we could identify in 10–60% of the patients cytokeratin-positive cells in bone marrow aspirates. Under conditions of nonmalignant disease, epithelial cells were absent in a group of 75 patients with various diagnoses, ranging from benign tumors to inflammatory diseases of the respective organs. In addition, a double staining of bone marrow with anti-CD45 antibody (leukocyte-common antigen) and anticytokeratin (18) antibody revealed a mutual exclusion of both markers on bone marrow cells; i.e., whereas nearly 100% of hematopoietic cells stained with anti-CD45, the very few (10^{-4} to 10^{-5}) cytokeratin-positive cells consistently lacked the CD45 antigen (Schlimok et al. 1987). Because the presence of such cells was correlated with the tumor staging in all three cancers tested, a further study of the nature of the disseminated cell was warranted. By applying a double-staining procedure with ^{125}I-labeled anticytokeratin antibody and alkaline phosphatase staining with antibodies against epidermal growth factor (EGF) receptor, transferrin receptor, the Ki67 nuclear antigen, and major histocompatibility complex (MHC) class I and class II common determinants, a rather heterogeneous picture emerged. In a group of patients with mammary carcinoma, the expression of EGF receptor, transferrin receptor, and Ki67 was analyzed in more detail. The expression of these markers on epithelial cells in bone marrow appeared to increase with tumor progression.

The question thus arose whether those cells exhibiting proliferation-associated markers could be propagated in vitro and whether they were tumorigenic in vivo. For this purpose, isolated nucleated bone marrow cells from patients with mammary, colorectal and gastric cancers were cultivated in RPMI medium with 10% fetal calf serum and several growth factors at various cell concentrations. The proportion of epithelial cells in the cultivated cells was monitored by staining the cell suspension at regular intervals with the CK2 anticytokeratin antibody. As shown in Table 1, an expansion of the epithelial cells was obtained in all three types of cancers tested so far. Although the primary inoculum was virtually free from epithelial cells, i.e., the frequency of cytokeratin-positive cells was on the order of 10^{-4} to 10^{-6} nucleated cells, epithelial cells grew out in a substantial proportion of bone marrow samples. Tumorigenicity of the cultivated epithelial cells was assessed after five to seven tissue-culture passages by transplanting the cells into nu/nu mice. The cells were injected by the subcutaneous, intraperitoneal, or intrahepatic route. Thus far, we have obtained two tumors with bone marrow from mammary carcinoma patients and one from a patient with colorectal cancer (Table 1). None of the three tumors was derived from patients with clinical visible metastasis (M_1); all three patients had been biopsied during surgery of their primary tumors. The tumor tissue exhibiting typical adenomatous histologic architecture was identified unequivocally as of human origin with

Table 1 Tumorigenicity and In Vitro Propagation of Epithelial Cells Isolated from Bone Marrow

Primary tumor[a]	No.	Multiplication in vitro[b]	Transplanted to nu/nu mice	Tumor growth
Breast cancer	18	8	8	2
Colorectal cancer	20	7	7	1
Gastric cancer	5	2	2	0

[a]Bone marrow was obtained from patients without overt bone metastasis.
[b]Yield of epithelial cells in vitro 4×10^4 to 3×10^6.

anti-MHC antibodies. It could be shown that from virtually disease-free bone marrow, epithelial cells can be expanded in vitro and assayed in vivo for tumorigenicity.

As reported previously, monitoring of epithelial cells in bone marrow of individual patients is feasible (Schlimok et al. 1987). The first clinical data after 31 months of observation show that mammary carcinoma patients presenting epithelial cells in their bone marrow are prone to relapse with a distinctly higher rate (81%), in comparison to those where epithelial cells were not found (11%). These data were obtained by a retrospective analysis of single-site aspirations in 89 patients.

Because multiple-site aspiration apparently increases the probability of detecting epithelial cells in bone marrow (Brunning et al. 1975; Dearnaley et al. 1983), we compared single-site with triple-site analysis. As shown in Table 2, in the group of patients without regional lymph node involvement (stage $T_{1-3}N_0M_0$), the percentage with positive bone marrow findings increases from 8.9% with single-site aspiration to 23.4% with triple-site biopsies. It is particularly this "nodal negative" group of patients that would benefit most from a more accurate assessment of their risk status. The more ag-

Table 2 Cytokeratin-positive Cells in Bone Marrow of Mammary Carcinoma Patients: Single- vs. Triple-site Aspiration

Stage	Single site		Triple Site	
	no.	%	no.	%
$T_{1-3}N_0M_0$	8/90	8.9	11/47	23.4
$T_{1-4}N_{1-3}M_0$	8/59	13.6	11/31	35.5

gressive and effective adjuvant chemotherapy could thus be reserved for those with a definite risk of relapse, whereas a larger low-risk group of $T_{1-3}N_0M_0$ patients could be spared from the toxic side effects of the current adjuvant treatment regimens. Thus, besides the monitoring of therapeutic effects, a better definition of risk groups could be of immediate clinical application in this new diagnostic procedure.

Tumor cells disseminated early from the primary tumor and successfully growing in the environment of a foreign organ must be regarded as a highly selected and successful cell population. The analysis of their growth characteristics and response pattern to environmental signals should yield new information on this critical period of tumor progression. In view of new therapeutic strategies, it is this stage of minimal tumor load now accessible for direct evaluation, which should be most amenable to immunotherapies involving antibodies, cells, or cytokines.

ACKNOWLEDGMENTS

This work was supported by Deutsche Krebshilfe and Wilhelm-Sander-Stiftung.

REFERENCES

Brunning, R.D., C.D. Bloomfield, R.W. McKenna, and L. Peterson. 1975. Bilateral trephine bone marrow biopsies in lymphoma and other neoplastic diseases. *Ann. Int. Med.* **82:** 365.

Dearnaley, D.P., M.G. Ormerod, J.P. Sloane, H. Lumley, S. Imrie, M. Jones, R.C. Coombes, and A.M. Neville. 1983. Detection of isolated mammary carcinoma cells in marrow of patients with primary breast cancer. *J. R. Soc. Med.* **76:** 359.

Debus, E., K. Weber, and M. Osborn. 1982. Monoclonal antibodies that distinguish simple from stratified squamous epithelia: Characterization on human tissues. *EMBO J.* **1:** 1641.

Schlimok, G., I. Funke, B. Holzmann, G. Göttlinger, G. Schmidt, H. Häuser, S. Swierkot, H.H. Warnecke, B. Schneider, H. Koprowski, and G. Riethmüller. 1987. Micrometastatic cancer cells in bone marrow: *In vitro* detection with anti-cytokeratin and *in vivo* labeling with anti-17-1A monoclonal antibodies. *Proc. Natl. Acad. Sci.* **84:** 8672.